THE COMPLETE ILLUSTRATED GUIDE TO
CRYSTAL HEALING

A Step-by-Step Guide to Using Crystals for Health and Healing

SIMON LILLY

Harper
Collins

HarperCollins*Publishers*
77–85 Fulham Palace Road,
Hammersmith, London W6 8JB

© 2002 by HarperCollinsPublishers Ltd
Text copyright © Simon Lilly 2002

www.harpercollins.co.uk

First published in 2002 by Element Books, an imprint of HarperCollinsPublishers Ltd.

1 3 5 7 9 10 8 6 4 2

Cover illustration © Rebekah Nichols/illoreps.com

Designed by quadrum▪
Quadrum Solutions, Mumbai, India
www.quadrumltd.com Tel: 91-22-24968210

A complete listing or picture credits can be found at the back of this book.

A catalogue record of this book is available from the British Library

ISBN 978-0-00-788545-9

Printed and bound in China by South China Printing Company Ltd

NOTE FROM THE PUBLISHER
Any information given in this book is not intended to be taken as a replacement for medical advice.
Any person with a condition requiring medical attention should consult a qualified practitioner or therapist.

Acknowledgments

To all our students, past and present, for their insight, patience and enthusiasm.

Contents

Introduction

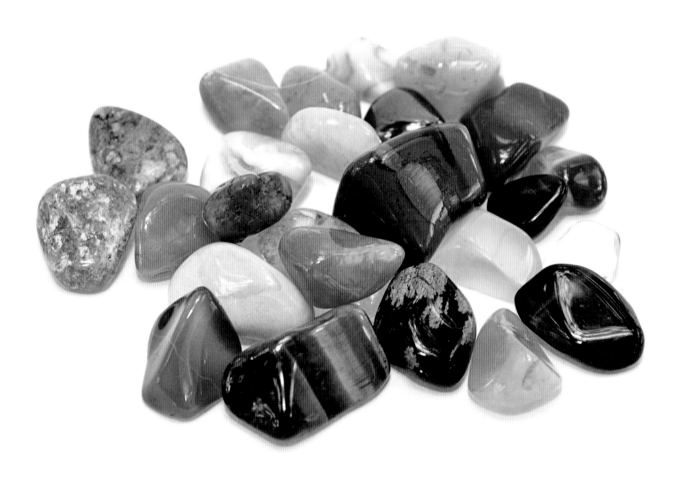

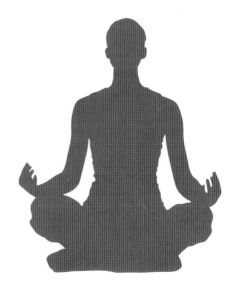

When we hold a crystal, we are instantly in touch with the forces that shape our planet and the elements that first formed eons ago in the heart of distant stars. Current scientific knowledge of the chemical structure and properties of crystals is comparatively recent. Scientific investigations into the properties of crystals have led to our present-day technological dependence on a variety of both naturally occurring and synthesized crystals. Our modern world would not be possible without such crystals. From computers to car engines, lasers to space shuttles, all have vital components that use these unusual bits of stone. The present-day interest in crystal healing is a continuation of humankind's constant fascination with gemstones and minerals throughout the ages.

ABOVE Crystals can balance, strengthen, and support the body's subtle energy systems.

In *The Complete Illustrated Guide to Crystal Healing*, I show the reader how to make use of crystals to enhance the body's own healing abilities, reduce stress, and improve the quality of life. There is no established system within the field of crystal healing yet, and in this book I have tried to cover those aspects of the subject that seem worthwhile and are accepted as standard practice. However, each therapist brings their own expertise and develops personal work methods. A distinction should be made between "healing with crystals" and crystal healing. Many healers use crystals as an amplification of their healing skills—as an adjunct to personal energy. Crystal healing—applying crystals in the right place at the right time—will initiate profoundly positive life changes. I hope this book will encourage experimentation with crystals to bring you lasting benefit.

BELOW Earth's riches: sparkling crystals formed from mixtures, liquids, or vapors in the Earth's crust.

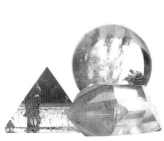

9

How to Use This Book

The Complete Illustrated Guide to Crystal Healing provides a unique survey of the history of crystal healing, as well as an account of the formation and structure of crystals. The basic procedures of crystal healing are explained, together with practical advice on choosing and storing crystals. The reader is encouraged to develop their intuitive skills using methods of assessment, such as pendulum dowsing and muscle-testing procedures. Descriptions of advanced healing layouts demonstrate how to balance the human body's subtle energy systems and ways to make crystals a part of everyday life by using them to enhance our surroundings.

RIGHT *The first part of the book will get you started by introducing simple healing layouts, which can help restore both energy and balance.*

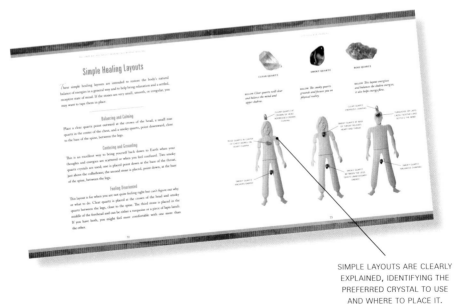

SIMPLE LAYOUTS ARE CLEARLY EXPLAINED, IDENTIFYING THE PREFERRED CRYSTAL TO USE AND WHERE TO PLACE IT.

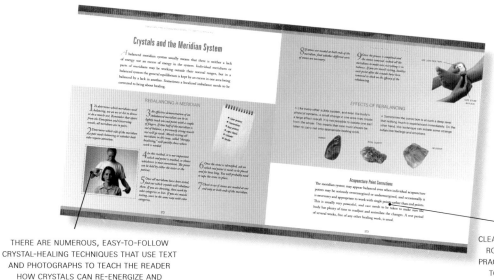

LEFT *The central part of the book clearly outlines the seven main chakras and the meridian system, detailing how particular layouts can strengthen and support these energy centers.*

THERE ARE NUMEROUS, EASY-TO-FOLLOW CRYSTAL-HEALING TECHNIQUES THAT USE TEXT AND PHOTOGRAPHS TO TEACH THE READER HOW CRYSTALS CAN RE-ENERGIZE AND RECHARGE THE BODY AND SPIRIT.

CLEAR TEXT GIVES A UNIQUE SURVEY OF THE ROLE OF CRYSTAL HEALING, AS WELL AS PRACTICAL ADVICE, FROM CRYSTAL LAYOUTS TO A DETAILED GEMSTONE DIRECTORY.

BELOW *As more advanced techniques are introduced, the reader is encouraged to explore the methods of crystal healing further.*

FIND OUT HOW TO DEVELOP INTUITIVE SKILLS BY USING DIFFERENT METHODS OF CRYSTAL HEALING.

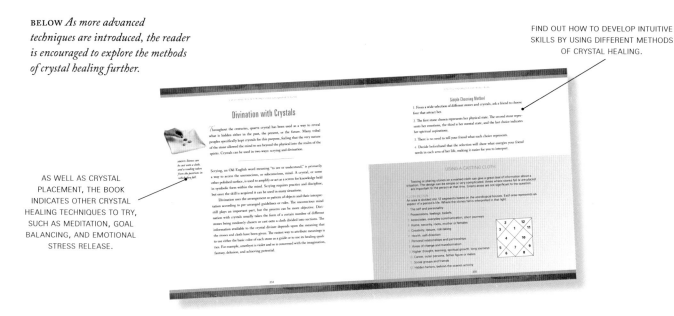

AS WELL AS CRYSTAL PLACEMENT, THE BOOK INDICATES OTHER CRYSTAL HEALING TECHNIQUES TO TRY, SUCH AS MEDITATION, GOAL BALANCING, AND EMOTIONAL STRESS RELEASE.

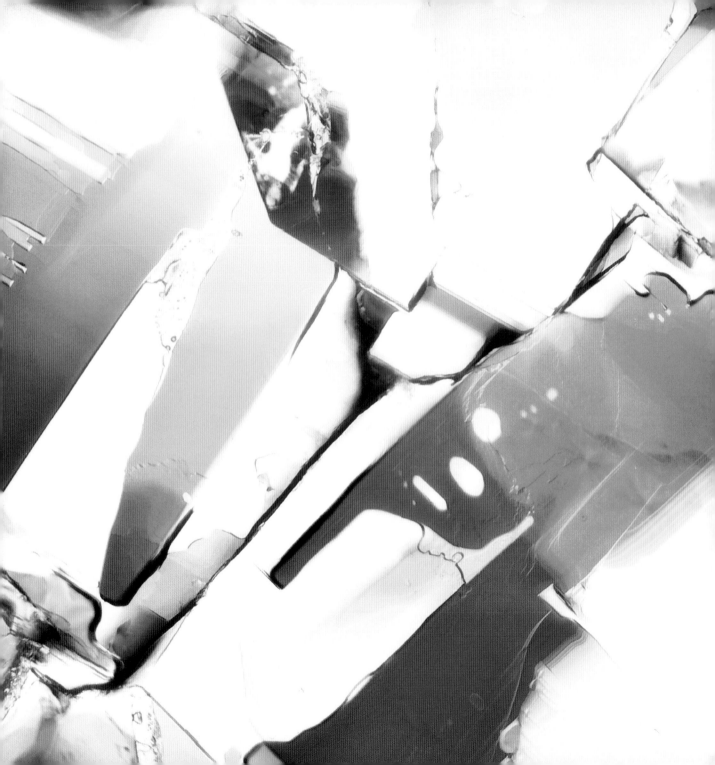

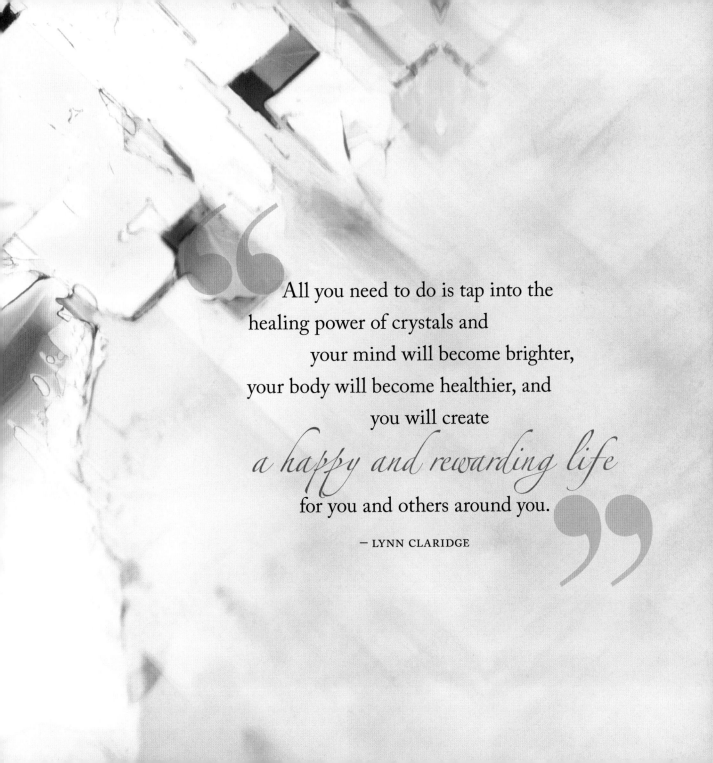

"All you need to do is tap into the
healing power of crystals and
your mind will become brighter,
your body will become healthier, and
you will create

a happy and rewarding life

for you and others around you."

— LYNN CLARIDGE

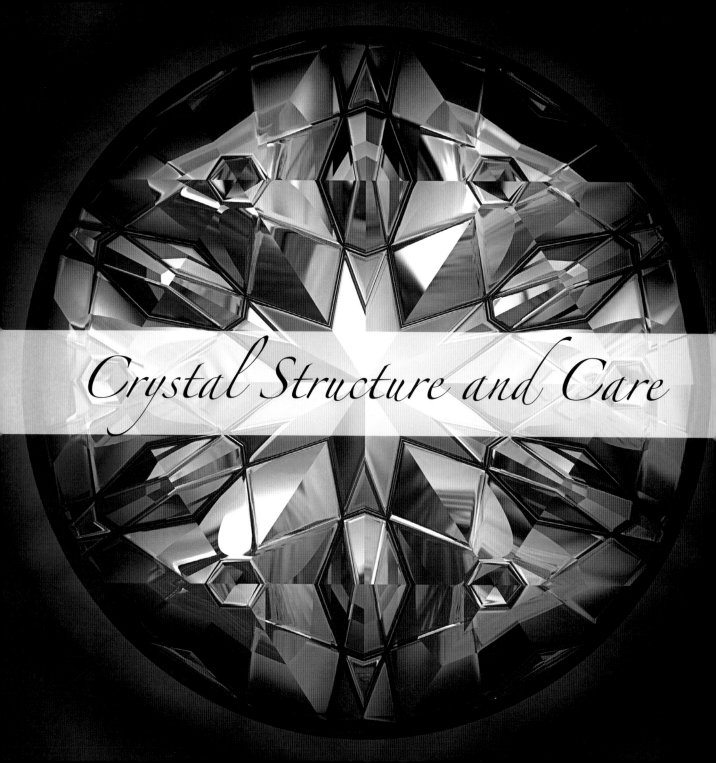

Crystal Structure and Care

Structure of the Earth

*I*t is important to place the mineral kingdom and its crystals in a larger context, in order to understand the unique properties of crystals and accept their use as a healing tool. The dynamics of continental drift, and the generation of heat and pressure deep within the Earth's crust, are the processes that lead to rock formation and crystallization.

The Earth is believed to be about 4.6 billion years old. From early in its existence, it is thought to have consisted of the same four layers that exist today: the outer crust, the mantle, and the outer and inner cores. It is nearly 8,000 miles (13,000 km) in diameter.

The outermost layer, the crust, is proportionately very thin. Under the oceans it is only about 5 miles (8 km) thick, increasing on the continents to an average of 20 miles (30 km) and, at its deepest, 55 miles (90 km) under the Himalayas. The crust makes up only 0.4 percent of the planet's mass! Nearly all the rocks in the crust are crystalline, and of these, the majority are formed of oxygen and silicon. The rest are composed primarily of six other elements—aluminum, iron, calcium, sodium, potassium, and magnesium.

The thin crust floats on the mantle—nearly 70 percent of the Earth's mass. The mantle is over 1,800 miles (2,900 km) thick and consists of different layers of swirling, very hot, thick melted rock called magma (lava). Little is known for certain of the core except that it comprises iron and nickel. The outer core seems to be liquid iron and nickle, while the inner core is thought to be solid iron.

ABOVE
The outermost layer of the Earth is the crust, where there are three types of rock: igneous, sedimentary, and metamorphic.

The Rock Cycle

Continental drift—the slow sliding of the massive tectonic plates that make up the Earth's crust—is responsible not only for making mountains as the continents collide, but also for creating many stress fractures, folds, and faults in the surface rock. This allows new material to well up from far below, changing the nature of many minerals through heat and pressure, while at the same time creating the perfect condition for new minerals to crystallize.

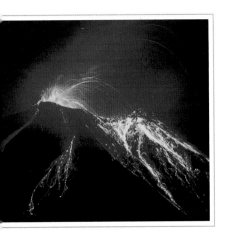

Plate tectonics is the engine that drives the continental process of rock formation and crystallization, which is known as the rock cycle. Understanding this cycle enables us to see how crystals are created and how the Earth's huge variety of minerals is made. Three types of rock are continually created by the processes of the rock cycle: igneous, sedimentary, and metamorphic.

Igneous rocks are formed when continental drift creates areas of stress deep in the Earth's crust. These cracks release some of the enormous pressure placed on the semifluid magma by the crust's moving plates. There is then a huge increase in temperature, liquefying the magma so that it flows upward through the cracks. If this super-heated, highly pressurized magma reaches the surface; it then either forms a volcano or spreads out as a lava flow. Sometimes the magma is stopped by a solid layer of rock so that it spreads out and then cools within the Earth. As the magma solidifies, well-defined crystals may form in hollow spaces, such as those left by gas bubbles. The majority of crystals are created from super-heated, mineral-rich gas and water, released as the rocks solidify. These solutions rise higher through crevices and cracks in the rock, crystallizing wherever the conditions of temperature and pressure are right. Depending on the elements in the solution, different crystals will grow.

ABOVE *Igneous rock starts off as hot liquid rock called magma, deep in the Earth's crust. Pressure can push it upward, and when it reaches the Earth's surface, it is known as lava.*

Metamorphic rocks have been changed from their original state by heat, pressure, or both. Existing rocks close to an igneous intrusion may be altered by a high local temperature that can drive off elements or add some new ones. Other metamorphic rocks are created by pressures within the crust. The types of crystals found in these rocks will depend on the original material and the metamorphic conditions.

Wherever rock reaches the surface of the planet, it will be eroded by wind, water, and temperature changes. Debris from this rock may be deposited far from its original site, and over millions of years thick layers build up and are gradually compressed to form new rocks. Crystals within these sedimentary rocks tend to be soft because they form at much lower temperatures and pressures, but they crystallize very rapidly and can create huge deposits of, for example, calcite and halite (rock salt). Sedimentary rocks are also subject to metamorphosis. Limestone, for example, turns into marble under heat and pressure.

BELOW *The rock cycle of change: rocks are pushed up, eroded, transported, compressed, and sometimes metamorphosed.*

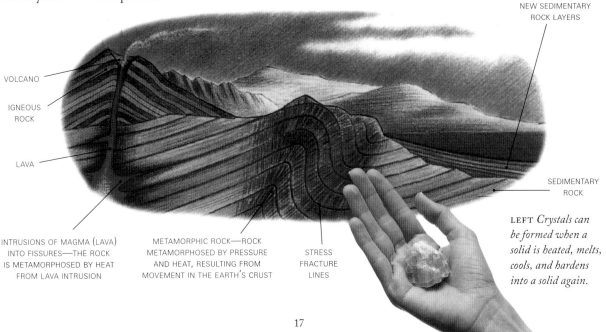

NEW SEDIMENTARY ROCK LAYERS

VOLCANO

IGNEOUS ROCK

LAVA

SEDIMENTARY ROCK

LEFT *Crystals can be formed when a solid is heated, melts, cools, and hardens into a solid again.*

INTRUSIONS OF MAGMA (LAVA) INTO FISSURES—THE ROCK IS METAMORPHOSED BY HEAT FROM LAVA INTRUSION

METAMORPHIC ROCK—ROCK METAMORPHOSED BY PRESSURE AND HEAT, RESULTING FROM MOVEMENT IN THE EARTH'S CRUST

STRESS FRACTURE LINES

Crystal Structure

A crystal is defined by its internal structure, which directly influences its exterior form. It is made up of atoms that have bonded together into regular, repeating patterns, and it is these patterns that create a crystal's solid form with flat faces, which are arranged in a precise geometry. This repeating pattern is known as a crystal lattice.

Crystals can form only from a gas or liquid solution because only in this state are atoms free to arrange themselves into stable relationships with each other. Depending on what elements are combined within the gas or liquid solution, different types of atoms will bond together into mineral crystals.

A crystal will always have the same fundamental internal order of atom structure lattices, no matter what it looks like—whether it is perfect, misshapen, battered, chipped, or eroded, or if it is perfectly clear, cloudy, or colored. A crystal lattice is built up very rapidly when one or two atoms take up a set pattern of bonding together. The shape of the original molecule, dictated by the size of the atoms of the elements involved, establishes the unit cell that is the smallest part of the crystal lattice. Other atoms of the same elements are attracted to this cell, and so the crystal builds up layer upon layer of repeating parts.

When all the available elements have been used, or when temperatures and pressures change in the surroundings, the crystal's growth stops, leaving its outermost atoms as flat external faces. The speed at which the liquid flows and the space available for growth tend to create distorted shapes, so that some crystal faces become larger than others. Every crystal is unique in appearance, but the angle between corresponding plane faces will be the same in all crystals of the same substance and structure. It is often possible to identify a mineral according to the shape of its crystals and the way that the crystallization has taken place. A single crystal can vary in size from a minute, submicroscopic particle to a mass as much as 100 feet (30 m) long.

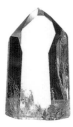

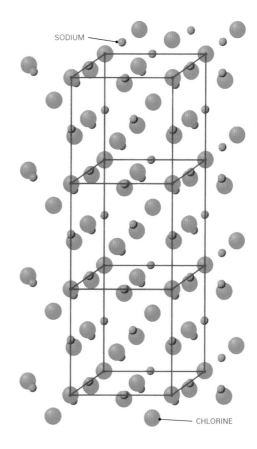

SODIUM

ABOVE *The external shape of a crystal, its flat sides and characteristic facets reflect the inner structure of its atoms.*

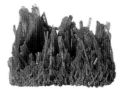

ABOVE *In rock crevices, crystals can only develop faces in the open space of the center of the cavity. This produces a crust of crystals lining a rock cavity, called a druse.*

CHLORINE

LEFT *The atomic structure of a salt crystal, showing the repeating geometric arrangement known as a crystal lattice.*

Unique Properties of Crystals

When a crystal grows, the lattice is very rarely perfect. Sometimes there are gaps in the structure, sometimes extra atoms are squeezed in, or an atom of a slightly different size enters the lattice. This means that, although it is in a state of equilibrium, the crystal has a reservoir of extra electrons. Because they are not all used up in the making of bonds between atoms, some electrons have nothing to do. When energy is put into the crystal, these electrons become excited and begin to flow through the lattice structure. This means that crystals can act as transducers, changing one form of energy into another.

One possible effect is that light energy may stimulate the electrons to become conductors, thus generating an electric current. Heat can create the same effects. Sometimes heat or friction will produce light in a crystal—pieces of quartz when rubbed together in a dark room will show triboluminescence. A sugar cube crushed in darkness will display flashes of green light. This is called piezoelectricity and happens when a crystal lattice is deformed

RIGHT
Piezoelectricity is utilized in quartz watches. The watch battery causes the quartz crystal to expand in regular pulses, thus driving the watch mechanism.

CRYSTAL STRUCTURES

• A crystal is a mineral in its most stable form.

• A crystal has a recognizable internal structure made up of repeating arrangements of atoms, known as a crystal lattice.

• The geometrical form of a crystal, with symmetrically arranged plane faces, is an expression of its internal atomic structure.

• Every crystal of the same mineral will have flat faces meeting each other at identical angles.

• Crystals are the most organized and stable matter in the universe.

• Crystals can grow to a huge size or appear as microcrystalline masses, where each crystal is too small to be seen with the naked eye.

• Crystals will only form from a gas or liquid solution at the correct temperature and pressure.

• Once crystallized, a mineral can remain unchanged for millions of years.

• Subjected to extreme conditions of heat and pressure, a crystal may alter its form or become another mineral altogether.

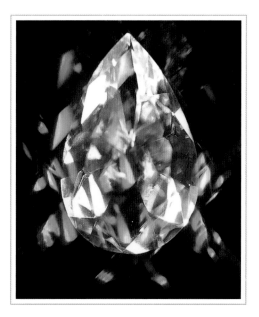

LEFT *A macrograph of a cut diamond, showing the exceptional light dispersion emanating from the crystal. Diamond is the hardest known mineral; it is the structure of its atoms that make it unique. This crystal is invaluable for industry because it is hard but very lightweight compared to steel, making it perfect for grinding, shaping, and cutting.*

enough to create a large electric current or an electric current deforms the lattice structure.

Another interesting possibility is that pressure in the form of sound may create unique electron excitement in a crystal structure, leading to the entrainment or storing of a word, phrase, or event. The perceived atmosphere of a place may be caused by the local crystal-bearing rock, or even the crystal-like structure of a body of water, retaining a pattern, imprint, or a memory of events. Within the structure of each crystal lattice, there are vortices and currents of energy held in place until some kind of extra input allows them to manifest in energetic guises. Today, solid state physics is beginning to reveal the mechanisms that healers and sensitives have subjectively experienced for millennia.

The Crystal Systems

$\mathcal{T}$here is a maximum of 14 different ways in which points can he arranged in space. These correspond directly to seven main crystal systems. Each system contains minerals whose constituent atoms have been arranged into regular lattices that have the same axes of symmetry in the same relationship to each other. This means that all of the crystals within a group tend to have similar basic shapes.

HEALING GEOMETRY

CUBIC SYSTEM

Crystals of the cubic system have all axes of symmetry at right angles to each other. The cubic system is noted for the qualities of foundation and stability and can be used where structural and physical repair are needed in the body systems. Their solidity and simple symmetry help organize things in a straightforward, clear manner. This system is the only one of the seven that does not distort or alter light rays as they pass through. It leaves everything as it is and so can be of great value in exploring the reality of a situation. Examples of the cubic system include gold, diamond, copper, fluorite, halite (rock salt), sodalite, garnet, and pyrite. No matter what other properties these stones exhibit, they will always be anchored at the level of practical reality.

TETRAGONAL SYSTEM

Crystals of the tetragonal system have all axes of symmetry at right angles to each other, but here one axis is longer. These crystals are associated with balancing and working well with opposites. Tetragonal crystals can be both absorbing and reflecting. Many can absorb unbalanced or negative vibrations and transmute them into life-supporting energy. Crystals of this system tend to grow as short prisms based on the three-sided pyramid of the tetragon. Examples are rutile, zircon, and apophyllite.

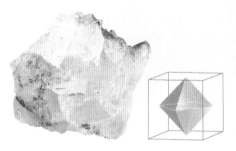

CUBIC SYSTEM

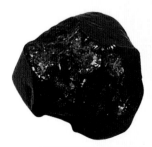

TETRAGONAL SYSTEM

Despite the difficulties in measuring and identifying the geometrical systems of crystallography, it is important to recognize that a crystal's geometrical form is the essence of why it does what it does, both in terms of its physical properties and its potential for healing.

Every physical object follows geometrical laws and is built upon three-dimensional patterns. Crystals are clear evidence for this fundamental organization of matter. Every crystal in a system will share certain energetic properties and ways of working. Like a crystal's color, its symmetry provides another method by which a stone's potential can be assessed.

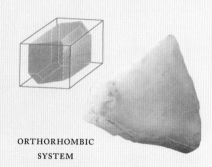

ORTHORHOMBIC
SYSTEM

ORTHORHOMBIC SYSTEM

The orthorhombic system has three unequal axes at right angles making prismatic or tabular crystals. They can be useful for bringing perspective and focus, and clearing away unnecessary patterns and unwanted energies. Orthorhombic crystals have a protecting, encompassing quality to them in which purification and cleansing can safely take place. Examples are peridot, topaz, sulfur, celestite, danburite, and staurolite.

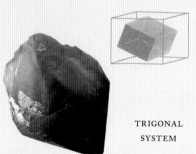

TRIGONAL
SYSTEM

TRIGONAL SYSTEM

The trigonal system is sometimes included with the hexagonal system. It has the same angles as the hexagonal but is made up as rhombohedral and triangular prisms. These crystals continually radiate energy useful for balancing the body's subtle anatomy, particularly where lack of energy is the problem. Trigonal crystals are more dynamic and focused in their activity than the hexagonal. Examples include agate, amethyst, bloodstone, carnelian, calcite, rhodochrosite, tourmaline, ruby, and sapphire.

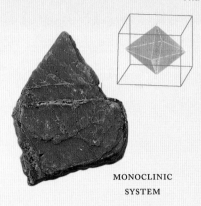

MONOCLINIC
SYSTEM

MONOCLINIC SYSTEM

The monoclinic system has three unequal axes, two at 90 degrees and one greater than 90 degrees. It forms various shapes but often has long prisms. In them, there is a continual expansion and contraction, a constant pulsing, that is stabilizing but encouraging to activity on some level. Monoclinic crystals are directional and can clear away obstructions. Clarity on deeper levels of perception can result from their cleansing action. Among the monoclinic crystals are azurite, jade, malachite, moonstone, selenite, lepidolite, amazonite, and kunzite.

HEXAGONAL SYSTEM

The hexagonal system comprises forms with three angles at 120 degrees and often appears as six-sided prisms and pyramids. Hexagonal crystals are characterized by growth and vitality. They emanate energy that may be used in healing, energy balancing, and communication. They help focus on particular areas of need and develop creativity and intuition. Useful as meditation and self-development stones, crystals of this system include emerald, aquamarine, quartz, and apatite.

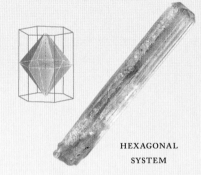

HEXAGONAL
SYSTEM

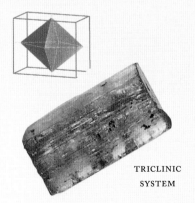

TRICLINIC
SYSTEM

TRICLINIC SYSTEM

The triclinic system has three unequal axes of symmetry, none the same as any other. This produces variable crystal forms, notably tabular ones. These crystals naturally tend to integrate different states of energy. They help merge and harmonize polarities where there is loss of balance. This can be of particular use in situations when beliefs and attitudes give rise to personality problems. Triclinic crystals can often work as vehicles to access different states of consciousness and finer, nonphysical dimensions. Crystals found in the triclinic system include turquoise, rhodonite, sunstone, labradorite, ulexite, and kyanite.

Choosing and Storing Crystals

*M*any people become interested in crystal healing because one or two stones or crystals attracted their attention as simply beautiful or interesting objects. Some people collect a few crystal clusters to decorate their homes, while others become fascinated with their variety of shapes and colors. It is easy to find yourself with a growing collection of rocks and crystals of all shapes and sizes.

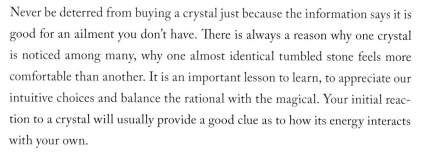

ABOVE *You are likely to find that you have a natural affinity with certain crystals.*

Never be deterred from buying a crystal just because the information says it is good for an ailment you don't have. There is always a reason why one crystal is noticed among many, why one almost identical tumbled stone feels more comfortable than another. It is an important lesson to learn, to appreciate our intuitive choices and balance the rational with the magical. Your initial reaction to a crystal will usually provide a good clue as to how its energy interacts with your own.

Pay special attention to those stones that are very attractive to you because they will probably be ones that are in tune with the current state of balance and energy within your body. Similarly, notice those stones that you instinctively dislike, since these will often represent qualities of energy with which you can't cope at the moment but will need to adjust to in time, or ones that begin a release of stress that creates a feeling of unease or discomfort in you as it occurs. The following guidelines may help you build a working collection of beautiful stones for use in healing and self-development.

Specimen Samples

Mineralogical specimens are usually fine and interesting examples of minerals in native bedrock. These can be large or delicate and are not easily used in healing situations, but they can add great energy and atmosphere to a room.

Natural Single Crystals

These are crystals that have been separated from their matrix and from any surrounding crystals but have not been worked or altered.

Worked Crystals

The most common form of worked gemstones can be found either in jewelry or in gem and mineral stores in the form of polished or tumbled pebbles of semiprecious stones.

Tumbled stones, which look like river pebbles worn smooth by water, are made by taking damaged crystals or large, broken pieces of stone and then placing them in revolving drums of grit for many days until they become smooth and polished.

Single large crystals that are slightly chipped or have a rough surface are sometimes repolished or ultrasonically cleaned to reveal their internal clarity.

Massive crystalline lumps may be carved or shaped into decorative statuary or natural-looking crystal shapes and tools such as massage wands *(see pages 195–197)* and spheres *(see page 184).*

RIGHT *A compartmentalized tray is the best way to store crystals, keeping the collection organized and protected.*

THE BASIC SET

Consider acquiring the following as a basic working set for crystal healing:

TUMBLED STONES can be found in a great variety of minerals. Select stones that are not too heavy or small. Bear in mind that you will need at least two stones of each spectrum color, although they can be different minerals.

SMALL, NATURAL CRYSTALS of clear quartz do not have to be large: 1¾ inches (2–4 cm) in length is fine. Twelve or more small quartz crystals is a good number to consider having.

SMALL, SINGLE CRYSTALS of amethyst quartz, smoky quartz, and citrine quartz are also worth looking for.

SMALL, HAND-SIZE CLUSTERS of clear quartz, amethyst, or other quartz varieties are very useful for recharging and cleansing your other stones and crystal jewelry.

LARGER, SINGLE CRYSTALS or tumbled stones that are easy to hold in your hands make very good tools for meditation and other self-development work. These will be special, personal crystals that you will feel intuitively drawn to.

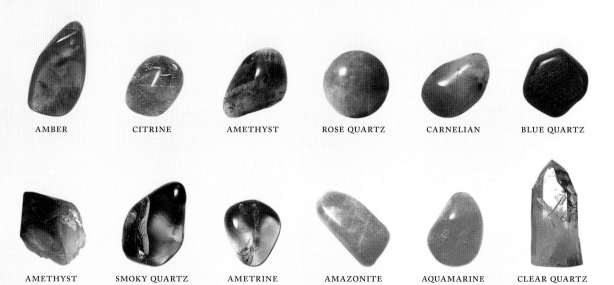

| AMBER | CITRINE | AMETHYST | ROSE QUARTZ | CARNELIAN | BLUE QUARTZ |

| AMETHYST | SMOKY QUARTZ | AMETRINE | AMAZONITE | AQUAMARINE | CLEAR QUARTZ |

Buying Crystals

If you are not lucky enough to have a selection of stores in your area that supply gemstones, check the jewelry stores. Many have small selections of tumbled stones and inexpensive cabochons and cut stones, often at a lower price. (A cabochon is a stone cut in a convex form and highly polished but not faceted.)

Storing Crystals

It is important to remember that even hard stones can be damaged by careless handling. Tumbled stones are the most robust because they have no delicate faces. Crystals, on the other hand, have tips and corners and are prone to chips and scratches if knocked together. It is a good idea to keep hard and soft stones separate to avoid damage. Be aware of which stones will fracture easily. Fluorite and calcite, for example, will readily shatter if dropped. Some crystals—especially the softer varieties such as halite, (rock salt) and selenite, a variety of gypsum—are very sensitive to humidity and may disintegrate completely in very damp conditions. Some, such as amethyst, may fade or change color if exposed to strong sunlight for long periods. Even quartz may shatter if internal flaws are exacerbated by rapid changes of extreme temperature.

If you own a crystal that is undamaged and perfect, remember that it may have been this way for many millions of years and treat it with care. However, many crystals do have chips, scratches, or rough surfaces. Whatever a crystal may look like, the internal structural harmony is the same for each example of that mineral. Some people choose the finest examples, others are happy with battered stones that are full of character.

An old printer's box, tool box, or fishing tackle box that has a lot of different-size compartments is ideal for storing your healing stones. Small pieces of foam or tissue paper can protect more delicate pieces.

Cleansing Crystals

*I*f you do not cleanse your healing stones, they will lose their efficacy and may even pass on imbalances to someone else the next time you use them. It is therefore vital you ensure that cleansing your crystals becomes an automatic process at the end of every healing session. There are many different cleansing methods; as with everything else, experiment and find the one you are most comfortable with.

Before and after you use a stone, it is a good idea to cleanse it in some way. If the stone is new to you, a simple wash in soapy water will help remove physical grime, fingerprints, and so on. Make sure the stone is not water-soluble (see Gemstone Directory)! Even more important is to remove any energy imbalances the stone may have picked up. Crystals have a tendency to absorb emotional stress and other strong energy patterns. Given time, a crystal will be able to restore its own internal equilibrium and neutralize the unwanted energy, but in a stress-filled environment the opportunity for rebalancing may not occur so readily. A crystal that needs cleansing may give the impression or feeling dull, heavy, or unpleasant. Regular cleaning is essential when crystals have been used for either healing or meditation. If you do not cleanse your healing stones, they will become less effective and may pass on their accumulated imbalances to someone else the next time you use them. Crystal cleansing should become a routine and automatic process after each healing session.

There are many different ways to clean your crystals. Try out these methods and use those with which you feel most comfortable.

ABOVE *Hold the crystals in the smoke from burning aromatic herbs in order to purify them.*

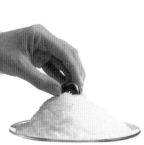

ABOVE *Salt absorbs imbalances and negativity.*

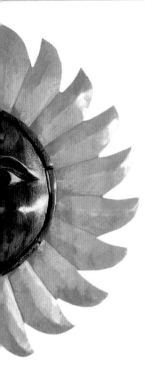

Sun and Water Method

Hold the stones under running water for a minute or so and then put them in the sun to dry. You could hold the stones in both hands and imagine all imbalances being washed from the stone, flowing away with the water. Or while the water is running over the stones imagine light gradually filling up the crystal until it is completely clear. A cloth or colander in the bottom of the sink will prevent breakage or loss down the drain.

This is an excellent method of cleansing newly acquired stones that are not water-soluble. However, if you have a lot of stones to cleanse, it can be a little tedious. A window ledge is fine if you don't have access to a safe spot outside, out of the way of pets and small children.

The Salt Method

Salt itself is a crystal used for centuries as a preservative and protector from negativity. Salt has the ability to draw imbalances into itself, so if you use

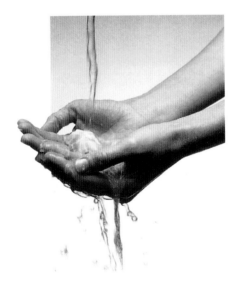

ABOVE AND RIGHT *Let the natural energies of water and sunlight cleanse the crystals after a healing session before you use them again.*

this method always throw away the salt afterward. Some people suggest using salt water, but this is only appropriate with harder crystals (it will damage and dull softer stones). Even with crystals such as quartz, it is difficult to wash away the salt from the little cracks and crevices, where it will recrystallize. The easiest method is to bury each stone separately in dry sea salt. Leave them for about 24 hours, then wipe the stones carefully.

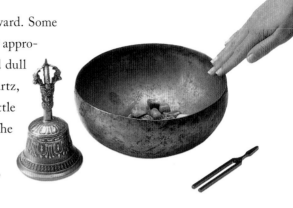

Incense Smoke

Herbs such as frankincense, sandalwood, sage, and cedar have a long traditional use in purification rites. Any aromatic smoke will help clean crystals that are held in the smoke. Solid incense, incense sticks, or smudge sticks will all work well.

Crystal Clusters

Placing single stones on a large crystal cluster will help. Crystal jewelry can be left on the cluster overnight. Alternatively, surround a stone with clear quartz crystals, points toward the center, and leave for 24 hours.

Sound

The vibrations of pure sound can quickly clean a stone. A singing bowl, one made of metal alloy that resonates when struck or rubbed along the rim, is very useful because it can hold many stones at once and will clean stones thoroughly and quickly in a minute or so. The sound will also have a purifying effect on the surroundings. A bell, gong, or tuning fork can also be used. Sound them close to the crystals until they feel completely cleared.

ABOVE *The vibrations of sound waves will wash the crystals clean.*

Visualization

Visualization can be useful where other techniques can't be used. Experimenting will help you choose which works best for you. The imagery is less important than your clarity of intent. Fill the stone with bright light, visualize water rushing through the stone or fire burning away all impurities, or imagine the stone as an animal shaking water off its fur after swimming. Use your breath to heighten the imagery. Take a deep breath, pause, and then forcefully blow over the crystal. As you do this, imagine all negativity clearing away from the stone. Repeat this until you feel it has worked.

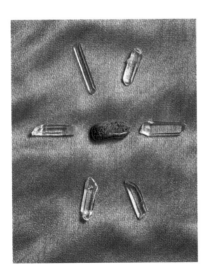

ABOVE *Surround the used stone with a pattern or circle of quartz crystals.*

BELOW *Use mind power to visualize imbalance being removed from each stone in turn.*

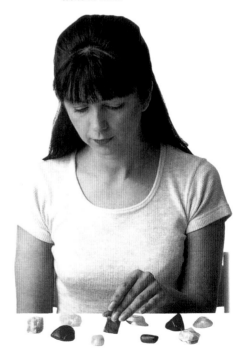

Gem Water and Gem Essences

*T*he unique properties of water mean that it is possible to make simple, effective essences of enormous value to healing processes. A gem essence is essentially a liquid version of a gemstone's energy patterns, and because it is liquid it can be used in ways that the stones themselves cannot. It is a simple matter to make your own gem essences, but be aware that some minerals are toxic and should be avoided.

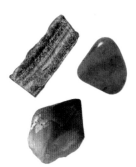

It is thought that the particular atomic bonding between the hydrogen and oxygen atoms in a molecule of water allows much greater range of movement than in other substances. This means that water can hold a memory or an energy pattern of something placed within it.

ABOVE *These stones are all members of the quartz family and are safe for making gem water.*

Toxic Stones

It is important what sort of stone is used for making gem water, particularly if you intend to drink it. Be aware that some minerals are toxic and should be avoided. The quartz family is sufficiently hard and is nontoxic and has such a

HEALING ENERGY

The potent water of these essences holds the energy characteristics of the gemstone. When this is brought into a person's subtle body, it encourages positive change, probably through the principles of resonance. The advantage of essences and gem waters is that they allow the body to balance itself at its own pace and will not usually bring about unnecessary changes. They help the body deal with the underlying stresses that may cause emotional or physical upsets.

great variety that a stone for most purposes can be found from a quartz selection. Softer stones tend to be more water-soluble than hard ones, so are more liable to form a chemical solution with possible toxic effects. If in any doubt, consult an expert or mineralogical textbook.

Keeping one or two clear quartz crystals in a water pitcher enhances the beneficial effects of the water. Try gem waters with different types of quartz—for example, clear quartz, amethyst, tiger's eye, or aventurine—and see how the taste varies!

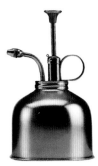

BELOW *Use a diffuser to spray pets and plants with gem water to keep them in good health.*

Gem Water

It is simple to make your own gem water (see right for ideas on use).

• Put a cleansed sample of a gemstone or crystal in the bottom of a clean, plain-glass tumbler or pitcher.

• Fill the tumbler with fresh water—spring water, if at all possible.

• Leave for 10–12 hours or overnight—it is best to use water immediately, although you can store it in the refrigerator.

SUGGESTIONS FOR USE

Gem essences and waters are excellent for self-help, and there are many ways of using them.

• Adding a couple of drops of gem essence to bath water will mean that the whole body and its subtle energy fields absorb the remedy very rapidly.

• Put a few drops into a diffuser sprayer with water and then spray it around the body. This will really change the energy feel of a place and is a useful way to cleanse a space or change its mood. Spraying pets and plants can help maintain their health in a simple way. Pets and plants will also benefit from being given gem water to drink once in a while.

• A couple of drops can be rubbed into the hands, then inhaled or passed around the body to cleanse the aura.

• Rub a drop into the body's pulse points, such as the wrists, throat, and forehead.

• Add three or four drops to a glass of water and sip it throughout the day.

• Place a couple of drops under the tongue once or twice a day.

GEM ESSENCES

Gem essences are made in a slightly different way and have the advantage of a longer shelf life than gem water. They use the energy of sunlight to activate the memory of water.

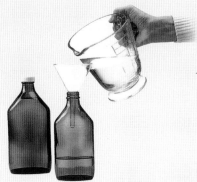

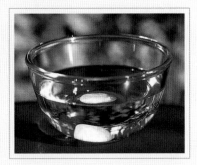

1 *Place a clean sample of crystal in the bottom of an undecorated, plain glass bowl. Add spring water until it just covers the crystal.*

2 *Place the bowl containing the crystal in full sunlight, perhaps on a windowsill outside, for at least two hours.*

3 *Afterward, carefully pour the water into a storage bottle that contains at least 50 percent brandy or vodka to act as a preservative. If a dropper bottle is used, drops can be taken as necessary. This is known as the mother essence.*

4 *Put between three and seven drops of a mother essence into a clean dropper bottle containing a 50/50 mixture of water/brandy for regular use. This is called the stock bottle.*

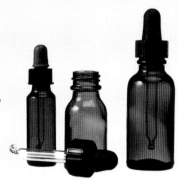

5 *If several essences are being combined, you can make one further dilution of a few drops from the stock bottle with 50/50 water/brandy. This is called a dosage bottle. If necessary, alcohol can be replaced with cider vinegar as a preservative.*

Varieties of Quartz Crystal

*C*lear quartz is the most common crystal used in healing. Every stone is unique in its shape and growth, but there are certain characteristic types that have acquired particular meaning for many who work with them. Quartz is a very coherent, resonant structure, and its outward shape tends to affect the less-organized structures around it, perhaps much more than another substance would.

Double-terminated Crystals

When quartz crystallizes in soft conditions of mud or sand, it is able to form terminations in more than one direction. Also, when crystals begin to grow on the sides of other crystals, they are able to extend far beyond their support, forming faceted points in both directions.

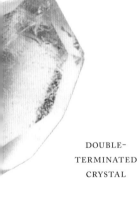

DOUBLE-
TERMINATED
CRYSTAL

These double-terminated crystals are able to move energy in two directions simultaneously and can act as a bridge between two energy points. They are used to help unblock negative energy. They have the ability to instill integration and poise and can make wonderful stones for holding during meditation.

Faceted Crystal

The size and the relationship of the facets reveal the sort of healing tool each crystal will be. The combination of shape and number carries great symbolic weight. A triangular face, suggests a very different energy characteristic than a seven-sided face, and so will be able to focus or channel energy in an entirely different manner. Ultimately, the usefulness of such categories must be determined by each individual healer.

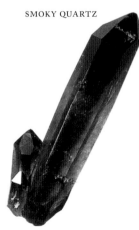

SMOKY QUARTZ

Herkimer Diamonds

Herkimer diamonds are a variety of quartz named after their original location in New York. Formed in cavities of soft, mudlike rock, they are generally small, very brilliant, double-terminated crystals of clear quartz. Herkimer diamonds concentrate and focus the qualities of light. This makes the stone very effective for cleansing toxins and blocks on many subtle levels of the body. The absorbent quality of Herkimer diamonds means that they will need regular cleaning to remain effective.

As a result of their multilevel rebalancing abilities, Herkimer diamonds have been found to amplify and improve subtle energy perceptions, clairvoyance, lucid dreams, and astral travel. Areas suffering from tension may well benefit from this stone.

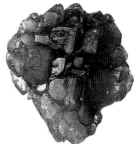

HERKIMER
DIAMONDS

Elestials

Elestials, or skeletal quartz, often take a peculiar form. They crystallize in a soft matrix, and natural terminations occur over large areas of the crystals, both on its sides and major facets, looking like steps or etched layers.

The key attribute of elestials is the revealing of hidden levels of situations or occurrences. They make useful personal meditation tools, both for holding and for looking at. They can help bring emotional stability, increase energy levels, and clarify expanded states of awareness. They tend to balance chakras *(see pages 118–124)* and subtle bodies *(see pages 151–152)*. Elestials can help link us more deeply to the forces of creation and reveal the underlying causes behind an illness or problem.

SMOKY QUARTZ
ELESTIAL

Tabular Crystals

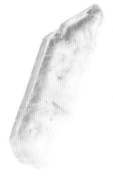

Tabular crystals form with two large flat planes, making a wide, thin crystal. They can often be double-terminated, and elestials may take a tabular form. This quartz crystal shape allows a rapid flow of energy to take place with little resistance. These stones facilitate communication between the levels within ourselves and other areas of creation. Confusion, misinterpretation, and misunderstanding can be alleviated by the use of tabular quartz. As meditation stones, they allow an easy flow of awareness to many areas of consciousness.

TABULAR QUARTZ

Scepter Quartz

This large crystal forms around the top of a quartz rod. These stones can direct healing processes to the center of a problem area, acting as both amplifier and a source of radiant energy.

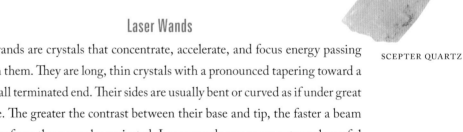

SCEPTER QUARTZ

Laser Wands

LASER WANDS

Laser wands are crystals that concentrate, accelerate, and focus energy passing through them. They are long, thin crystals with a pronounced tapering toward a very small terminated end. Their sides are usually bent or curved as if under great pressure. The greater the contrast between their base and tip, the faster a beam of energy from them may be projected. Laser wands can prove extremely useful for precision healing. If a tight beam of healing energy needs to be focused on a small area such as a meridian point, or to stimulate an area hidden within the body such as the pituitary or pineal gland deep in the brain, a laser wand is ideal. Wands can also remove extraneous debris from the subtle bodies, break harmful links to other people and things, and help isolate stubborn areas of imbalance. Laser wands are excellent amplifiers of intention, so great caution does need to be taken.

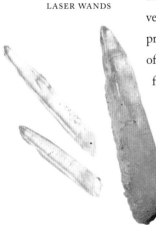

Intergrown Crystals

Where quartz crystals grow partly or completely surrounded by another larger crystal, they can express qualities of manifestation and protection. Small crystals can often be seen to grow a little way into the main quartz. This brings the quality of nurturing support and the development of new understanding about the relationship of inner and outer worlds to the crystal.

Much less common are whole crystals completely surrounded by another crystal growth. These stones make fascinating meditation tools; the enclosed crystal can represent aspects of the self. These stones also give effective protection from outside influences. They can also be helpful in bringing about wishes and desires. Here the intention is the interior crystal taking form on finer levels of reality and growing out toward the physical.

INTERGROWN
CRYSTALS

Phantom Crystals

Phantom crystals show the outlines and angles of earlier stages in their growth. Some phantoms are clearly visible, even opaque shapes seen within the transparent quartz. Others may be just the faintest of lines that resolve into planes when examined closely. The angles and shape of a phantom will always echo the final form of the crystal.

They make good meditation pieces and encourage the mind to dive to deeper levels of awareness. They can be helpful in tracing memories from long ago. In a healing context, phantom quartz can put past events into the correct perspective.

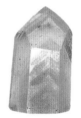

PHANTOM
CRYSTALS

Quartz Crystal Formations

Quartz crystals rarely grow in a perfect shape with six regular hexagonal sides meeting at a central point. The conditions of formation and environmental changes create a unique asymmetry and surface patterning. The size and shape of the resulting faces are thought to modify the sorts of energy each crystal can use.

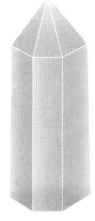

ABOVE *The generator yields an all-purpose energy.*

Generator Crystals

A generator quartz has six equal sides and six faces meeting together at the apex. They are very rare. Their general, all-purpose energy field positively charges spaces and acts as a focus for healing.

Transmitter Crystals

This form has two seven-sided faces with perfect triangular faces between them. This combination of seven-three-seven enables it to receive information and transfer it to the user, either from the Higher Self or another source. After grounding, centering, and attuning yourself to the crystal, clearly define your purpose or question. Then project this thought into the stone through a triangular face held to your brow. Leave the crystal in an upright position in a quiet place for a day. Sit with the crystal again and in a receptive, quiet state place the triangle to your brow chakra *(see pages 112–113)*, and absorb the information.

BELOW *Use the transmitter to receive and transmit information.*

Channeling Crystals

In this type of crystal, the largest face is seven-sided and is opposite a small triangular face. It can be used for meditation and for getting answers to specific questions. The large face of a channeling crystal helps access the intuition and can be held to the brow chakra or rubbed with the thumb. Where the crystal face is large enough, a channeling crystal makes a good tool for contemplation and scrying *(see pages 234–237)*.

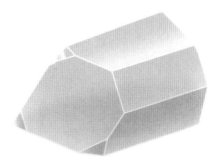

ABOVE *Channeling crystals are excellent aids to meditation, providing insight and inspiration.*

Occasionally it is possible to find a crystal that has characteristics of both transmitting and channeling crystals. These are known as trans-channeling, or Dow, crystals. They can be identified by their regular faces of equal proportions, with alternating seven-sided and triangular facets. Dow crystals are said to provide a continuous free flow of energy and information between all levels of creation and the self. These crystals can provide inspiration and a clear balancing environment and usually have a distinct personality.

Window Crystals

Many crystals exhibit small diamond or rhomboid faces between larger facets. Where the diamond is as large as other faces, with each angle joining the facet angles, it is known as a window crystal. Large window crystals are not common. The diamond shape symbolizes both clarity of mind and the ability to reconcile information from different levels of the mind.

Window crystals are mainly used to assess the energies of another person or to look inside oneself. This can be done by holding the window toward the

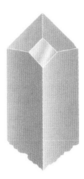
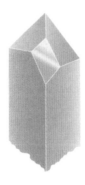

ABOVE *Window crystals with diamond and parallelogram facets encourage the mind to move through different levels of understanding.*

person for a while and then turning it to face the brow chakra, allowing the images and impressions to register on your conscious awareness. For working with yourself, gaze into the window with the intention of understanding the issue of concern. Again, place the window to your brow chakra and gather the impressions that come to you.

Where the window facet is not a regular diamond but a parallelogram, the quartz is sometimes called a time-link crystal. These crystals are used to shift awareness to different times, places, or dimensions. Some healers suggest a parallelogram skewed to the right will reveal futures, whereas one that leans to the left will view the past.

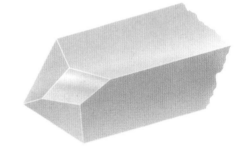

ABOVE *Window crystals reflect thoughts and inner energies: useful for assessing others and for self-awareness.*

Where a crystal has many parallelograms or a combination of diamonds and parallelograms, each acts as a doorway to different levels of reality. To work with a window crystal, ground and center your energies *(see pages 53–64)* and quieten your mind. Gaze without effort into the window, and when there is subtle awareness of a wavelike motion or pulsing, close your eyes and breathe in time with the sensation. With a clear destination in mind, focus your awareness just above the top of your head and let the mind travel. As with all of this kind of work, have a grounding stone nearby for your return to normal consciousness.

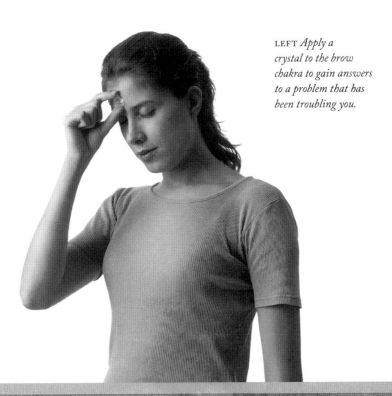

LEFT *Apply a crystal to the brow chakra to gain answers to a problem that has been troubling you.*

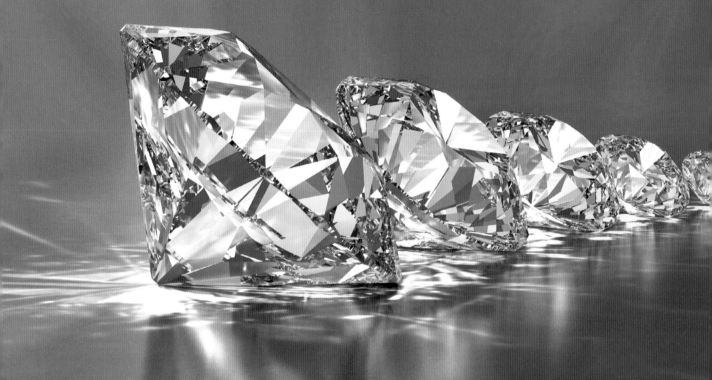

Crystals and Healing

Healing Power

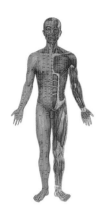

*T*here is no credible explanation as to why crystals and other gemstones should have any beneficial effect whatever on the human being from the point of view of Western medicine. Even though the properties of some minerals make possible the advanced technology that medical doctors use today, as well as being the raw materials with which pharmaceuticals are manufactured, there is no construct in mainstream science that allows for such an effect. It is only in the last few years that Western medicine has recognized that the emotions and the mind may play a part in the healing process. Traditional healers, however, have known this through their own experiences for thousands of years.

Explaining how crystal healing might work in terms of accepted Western science is not going to convince many people. However, it is possible to suggest by analogy how crystals might have such positive effects on the human body. Each crystal has one molecule, which is repeated throughout its structure. It has inherent order and the ability to adjust rapidly to all kinds of environmental changes. A crystal has a fundamental stability and, at the vibrational level, can maintain a constant electromagnetic signature.

The human body, on the other hand, is built up from thousands of different molecules, each with its own vibratory pattern and way of interacting with surroundings.

The simplest unit of the body—the cell—contains DNA and RNA, each with thousands of molecules, as well as proteins, enzymes, and internal structures. Each of these has different biomagnetic fields and electrical charges and belongs to larger and more complex systems.

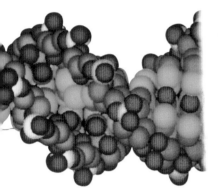

ABOVE *From its basis as DNA, the complexities of the human body encompass myriad systems and interactions.*

Imagine the body as a huge orchestra, with millions of individual instruments representing different vibrational signatures. The instruments are all using the same basic score—like the sequences of DNA—but are following their own parts—the function of the cell, organ, and system—and playing continuously without a break for a complete lifetime of 60, 70, or 80 years.

When the body is stressed, there is an alteration in the functioning of the whole system, and this is like one instrument going slightly off-key or falling behind the others, creating a small disharmony. Bringing a crystal into this cacophony of vibrations is like striking a tuning fork. One single, pure tone is emitted that can act as a guide by which members of the orchestra can retune their instruments and re-establish harmony.

Since crystals are, in fact, the simplest forms of matter, they may be seen to represent all possible combinations of energy and reflect the basic harmonies of nature. Because any state of disharmony within the individual is caused by a natural imbalance, the introduction of the appropriate stones or crystals into the energy fields of the body can help restore this harmony.

Wellness and Illness

The human being does not stop at the skin. Even orthodox science measures the thermal layer—equivalent to a planetary atmosphere—and a complex electromagnetic field generated by all the electrical and chemical processes in the body. This bioelectromagnetic envelope is extremely sensitive to all outside influences, which may only be registered subconsciously by the body.

Wellness can be understood as a stable state in which every energetic influence upon us can be utilized in a positive way, or neutralized easily. Illness occurs when other patterns that do not belong to our own nature are so much

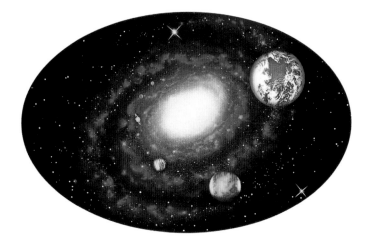

LEFT *The solar system is one small part of the energy signature of the galaxy. Today's quantum scientists suggest a theory of superstrings as the most fundamental of elemental particles, which somehow tie all existing forces of matter together and underpin all of creation.*

stronger than our own—and are in such contrast—that they begin to disrupt our characteristic field patterns.

Where there is slightly less order in a system through inherent weakness or stress of some kind, there will be a place where the imbalance will begin to show itself. In the body there are many types of potentially life-threatening bacteria and viruses that do not cause any apparent ill effects until a stress of some kind disrupts the equilibrium of the body, giving them the chance to proliferate and cause health problems. Health is a delicate balance between a multitude of factors.

Crystal healing does not concern itself primarily with physical symptoms or disease. From a holistic viewpoint, these are simply the tip of the iceberg. Removing the tip will not necessarily improve the situation. The majority of the problem is still there, and there is a distinct probability that it will resurface.

We can visualize these stress factors as a series of steps or levels, like sediments building up from an ocean floor. When overall stress rises to a certain height, it will appear above the surface. This is when symptoms of illness will appear. The symptoms will vanish once more if a therapy is able to reduce the amount of stress in one or more of these levels, thus reducing the total height.

A sudden increase in any one level, such as trauma or a buildup of environmental pollutants, may push us into a disease state. The form that the disease takes will very often be within the uppermost stress layer. If there is an underlying chronic infection of the throat, we will tend to get recurrent throat infections whenever the body is run-down. Effective healing can thus be defined as any system that releases enough stress from the underlying energy structures of the body so self-repair and self-regulation can be restored.

It is important to address the particular type of stress that each individual has acquired. If lifestyle is a major stress-creating factor, balancing meridians might reduce symptoms for a while, but the lifestyle stress will continue to dominate and increase. Removing stress from the lifestyle will reduce the overall stress-loading and is more likely to achieve lasting results.

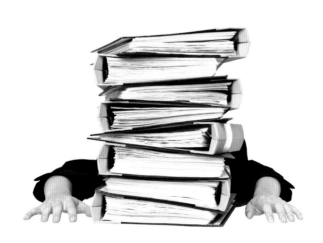

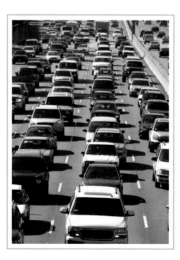

LEFT *Balancing your energies will not be nearly so effective if you are unable to reduce or avoid other stress factors in your life.*

Healing Session

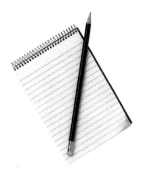

Crystal healing is a very individual therapy. Some healers may use crystals as an adjunct to massage or reflexology; others use crystals combined with spiritual healing. At the first session, the healer will take the patient's case history, asking about any serious illnesses, hospitalizations, and accidents, as well as current medicines or treatments. The healer may note any emotional or life trauma around the time of the illness.

ABOVE *Be prepared to give medical and lifestyle details to the healer.*

On the initial visit, many people find that it is the first time they have been allowed to fully describe their circumstances and feelings about their condition. A crystal healer, unless also a doctor, will not give any medical opinions but will offer support for the human and emotional aspects of the problems faced.

Before seeing the patient, the healer will have centered and grounded him or herself *(see pages 53–64)*, and may also have spent some time in prayer or meditation. All stones will have been cleansed and charged, and the working space cleared of all imbalances before healing can begin.

It is best to remove shoes and wear light, loose, comfortable clothing. The patient may be asked to remove any jewelry to ensure the body energies are not masked by other electromagnetic fields. The healer may now assess what healing work is a priority using techniques such as dowsing or muscle testing or intuitively scanning the person's auric field with a hand. Stones will be placed on or around the patient, or the healer may work with hand-held crystals *(see pages 179–182)*.

VISITING A CRYSTAL HEALER

INTRODUCTORY DISCUSSION

The first step in the crystal healing session will be some recording of case history; the healer will review the patient's current state of health and his or her past experiences. Sometimes, particularly where the patient is distressed, the healer might suggest that one or more crystals are held in the hand during the introductory conversation to bring calm and create an initial balance.

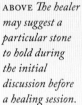

ABOVE *The healer may suggest a particular stone to hold during the initial discussion before a healing session.*

THE HEALING SESSION

During the first session and subsequent sessions, the healer will use specific crystals to balance the patient's chakras, energy centers, and other subtle systems in order to allow the experience of increased harmony to be programmed into the body.

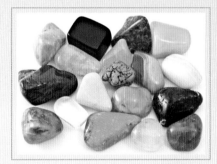

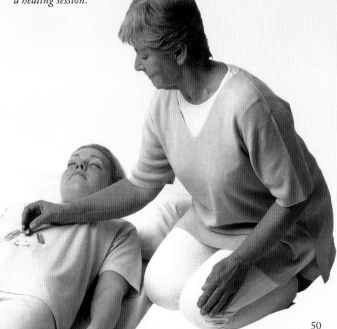

LEFT *Several techniques may be used in one session, or a single placement may be enough.*

AFTER THE HEALING SESSION

The healing might end with a brief discussion of what has been addressed. Further visits may be considered worthwhile, as crystal healing works best as a cumulative process. A crystal balance once a month for three or four visits will really help maximize the benefits in many cases. The healer might suggest a stone to carry or use at home, a gem essence to take, gem water to use, or may run through some simple exercises or meditations to help maintain energy balance between sessions.

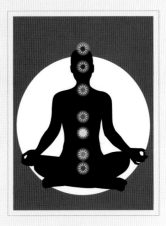

ABOVE *The seven chakras are the centers of the body and often the focus of healing sessions.*

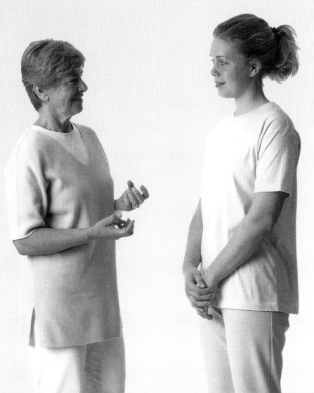

LEFT *The healing might end with a brief discussion of the energy work and any sensations the patient has experienced during the session.*

Some healers work in near silence or with gentle background music. Others ask for feedback to establish how the patient is feeling, whether there are any changes in perceptions or body sensations.

If the healer locates an area that needs a lot of work, the patient might be asked whether any physical symptoms have been noticed there, but the imbalance may never have reached a physical level. Most healers will appreciate the patient relating experiences of sensations, memory, or visual impressions received while stones are in place but will also understand if the patient is too deeply relaxed to communicate. Any feelings of discomfort or disorientation should be mentioned to the healer, as he or she can usually modify or ease them.

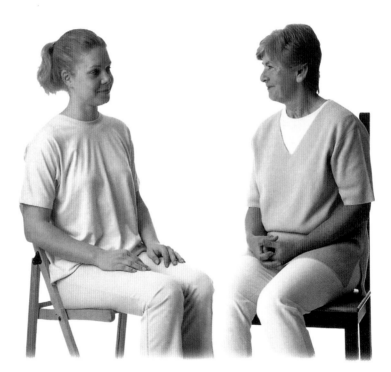

RIGHT *Discuss any recent emotional upsets so that the healer sees a complete health picture.*

Grounding and Centering

*O*f all the qualities needed to be an effective healer, perhaps the most important is that degree of focus and awareness that has become known as being centered and grounded. Grounding ensures that the healer is plugged into the correct power source and does not accumulate excess energy. Centering enables the healer to start any crystal work from a stable, clear base, to ensure that assessments are as accurate as possible.

BELOW *Being centered is like achieving a perfect balance through awareness of the body's center of gravity.*

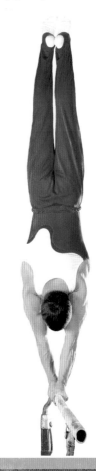

Grounding means being completely focused and present at all times. Subjectively, this is experienced as a feeling of solidity and security. There is a quality of mental focus and stillness and of having self-control in any situation. A lack of being grounded is experienced as nervousness, an inability to focus on the present, or to concentrate because of a wandering mind, or feelings of instability. When we are not grounded, energy either dissipates immediately or builds up to an intolerable level that may express itself as a loss of temper or restless discomfort. Being grounded means that all energy that passes through the body can remain in balance, with any excess flowing into the Earth, where it is safely dissipated. This helps prevent us from being overwhelmed or feeling dazed or disoriented—essential when using crystals as part of the healing process. Habitual lack of grounding leads to an imbalance of subtle energy, particularly in the chakra system, which can lead to burnout or health problems.

We are centered when all physical, mental, and emotional energies are integrated and balanced, bringing about a state of calm receptivity. To remain centered, there must be awareness of personal boundaries and the flow of energy.

Before and after every healing exercise, a healer should carry out a grounding procedure. The more they are practiced, the quicker the body recognizes when it is out of balance and the more effective any correction becomes. The process of healing requires working within someone else's states of imbalance. If healers fail to ensure their own equilibrium, they risk creating greater imbalance by inappropriate actions or taking risks and absorbing their patients' imbalances.

Being grounded means having a sound connection to planet Earth, and this creates a circuit of flowing energy and protection. Being fully aware within the body is one of the best protections from imbalanced energy of any kind. There are some people who habitually live in an ungrounded state, frequently equating their lack of focus with spirituality.

RIGHT *An effective grounding and centering technique involves visualizing a tree: imagine strong branches reaching upward, balanced by firm, healthy roots.*

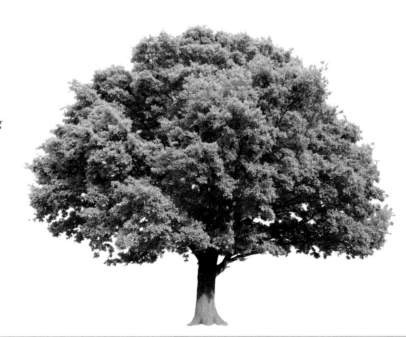

BASIC GROUNDING SET

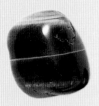 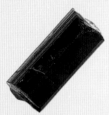 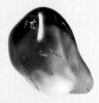 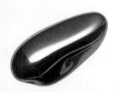

TIGER'S EYE	SCHORL	SMOKY QUARTZ	JASPER	HEMATITE
May have an attractive banded appearance.	Identified by its clearly striated sides.	Varies in color from smoky yellow to brown and black.	An opaque, usually red, yellow, or brown stone.	A dark, shiny mineral containing about 70 percent iron.

Passive Grounding Techniques

Little or no thought is required for passive grounding techniques, which makes them ideal when there is such a loss of balance that it is impossible to focus attention. There are several stones that can be used to ground one's energies effectively. Those included here work for most people, but there are always exceptions. Get to know which are most effective for you personally. In general, deep red, dark, and earthy colored stones will help focus energy within the physical body and reconnect it to the Earth.

Black tourmaline, sometimes called schorl, is a very good grounding stone and will also help protect from negativity. Smoky or black quartz can also work well. Minerals of iron, such as lodestone (magnetic iron ore) and hematite (iron oxide), are equally effective. Often more gentle in their action are stones like tiger's eye, iron pyrites (fool's gold), dark citrine quartz, and the dark red stones like garnet and jasper (red quartz) that will help ground by increasing physical energy.

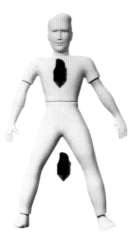

LEFT *Place smoky quartz crystals at the base of the throat and spine in order to collect thoughts and energies.*

The effect of grounding stones can be felt if they are held in the hands, worn, or placed near the body. If the stones have natural points, known as terminations, the technique is usually more effective if the points are facing down toward the ground. This encourages the grounding of energy. Likewise, putting the stone between the feet if seated, or below the feet, between the legs, or close to the base of the spine if lying down, encourages the base chakra and those grounding centers near the feet to balance body energies. Jewelry made with grounding stones will help keep a person grounded and protected, although ideally, other, more permanent methods (such as meditation or yoga) should also be learned.

Most forms of crystal healing will benefit from the addition of one or more grounding stones placed near the base of the spine or near the feet. These allow for the stabilization of any healing work carried out, so that changes can be more easily integrated permanently into the subtle energy systems of the human body. Without grounding stones, disorientation can occur and corrections may not last when the stones are finally removed.

Grounding Layout

This will ground and center in a couple of minutes:

• Place a smoky quartz crystal, point, downward, at the base of the throat.
• Place a second smoky quartz crystal at the base of the spine between the legs, with the point facing toward the feet.

Additional Exercises

Focusing attention on the physical body can be a useful way of becoming grounded. Any moderate activity or exercise, particularly if it is in contact with the Earth, will help.

• Take physical activities, such as walking, running, gardening, stamping your feet, or dancing.
• Eat or drink a little. Once the digestive system is occupied, a feeling of solidity returns.
• Sip a little cool water. Water helps speed up healing corrections by balancing the electrochemical systems of the body.
• Sipping a little hot, sweet tea or eating a piece of chocolate are also effective methods.

Attention Exercise

Breathe through a slightly opened mouth. Focusing on the roof of the mouth, notice that you feel the cool air as you inhale but no sensation when you exhale. Focusing on this for a moment or two helps calm the mind, centering awareness into the meridians of the body.

COOK'S HOOKUP

There is a useful technique derived from Kinesiology called Cook's Hookup, which will help both ground and center when energies are scattered. Because it integrates the left and right sides of the brain, this exercise reduces confusion and lack of coordination, as well as easing stress and upset. It is best to perform the exercise while sitting in a chair.

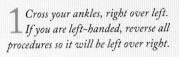

1 *Cross your ankles, right over left. If you are left-handed, reverse all procedures so it will be left over right.*

2 *Cross your wrists in front of you, right over left.*

3 *Now roll your hands so the palms are facing each other.*

4 *Interlace your fingers and then lay your hands on your lap.*

5 *Relax, close your eyes, and breathe easily. As you settle, your feelings or emotions may seem to intensify. This is part of the stress-releasing process, so simply let the feelings come and they will subside.*

6 *When you feel calm and restored to normal balance, unclasp your hands and uncross your ankles.*

7 *Now place your feet flat on the floor.*

8 *Rest your hands in your lap with just the fingertips touching each other as if you were holding a small ball between your palms. If you keep this position for half a minute, the benefits will last longer.*

HOLD FOR
30 SECONDS

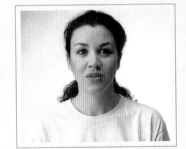

FINGERTIPS
TOUCHING

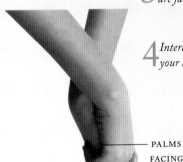

PALMS
FACING

INTERLACED
FINGERS

LEFT *Breathe through a slightly opened mouth*

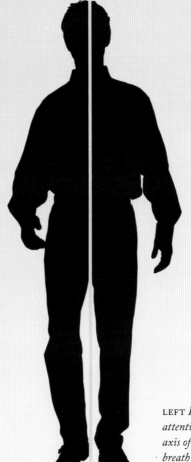

1 Imagine a line extending through your body from below your feet to the top of your head, positioned just in front of your backbone.

2 In your mind's eye, extend that line of energy down into the Earth as deep as you can go.

3 With each breath, imagine pulling energy up the line and into your body.

4 As you exhale, let your breath pass down into the Earth, each time you exhale pushing the line a little deeper toward the center of the Earth.

5 After a minute or two, move your attention to the top end of the line. Now, after you have drawn in breath from the Earth, breathe it out into the universe through the top of your head.

6 With your next breath, draw universal energy into the lungs and breathe it out into the Earth.

7 Continue this new cycle for a few minutes by repeating steps 5 and 6 so that you are alternately breathing in from the Earth and out into the universe, then in from the universe and out into the Earth.

8 You may find that your breathing automatically settles into a slightly different pattern. Don't worry if this happens.

9 When you have finished, relax, and take a moment or two to resume normal activity. With practice, you will be able to summon up this visualization whether you are seated, standing, or walking.

LEFT Focus your attention on the central axis of the body, using the breath to draw up energy along the midline.

Active Grounding Techniques

These grounding exercises are very effective, so long as you are able to do them without getting distracted. If you don't have enough focus, return to one of the more physically passive grounding techniques mentioned on *pages 55–56*.

When your energies feel scattered and have no direction and the mind is cluttered or racing, try any of the following imaging techniques:

Water Imaging Technique

Imagine yourself immersed under a waterfall or fountain. Completely surround yourself with the descending streams and imagine them also washing through you and then sinking deep into the Earth.

A more domestic image would be to imagine water faucets at the ends of your toes that you can turn on to drain away any excess energy, emotion, or tension into the Earth.

Breath Imaging Technique

Imagine that your breath is entering and leaving your body through the feet. When you inhale, draw the air up through the soles and send the exhalation out the same way. This will very quickly steady you because breathing deeper and more slowly than usual has a calming effect. The visualization illustrated on the next page uses breathing to help to focus attention on the central axis of the body.

Centering Techniques

A variety of different forms of meditation can be used for centering ourselves, although it is useful to discover those methods that create the desired result in only a few minutes. Focusing the attention on the breath can be very effective. Any simple yoga pranayama technique can be used.

Breathing Focus

Sit comfortably with your back upright. If support is needed, a firm cushion near your lower back will give great stability without restricting your breathing. Close your eyes and let your attention focus on the center of your chest. Take long, deep breaths through the nose. Continue for at least three minutes.

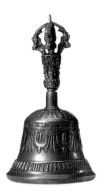

ABOVE *The clear tone of a bell quietens the mind.*

Sound Focus

Making use of sound can be a very quick way to return your body to a centered state. After settling down a little, by closing the eyes and taking a few slow, deep breaths, strike a tuning fork, bell, singing bowl, gong, or wind chime—anything that reverberates and gives a sustained, clear, and piercing sound when it is struck. Simply listen to the sound until it fades right away and is no longer perceptible. Continue sounding the note until you feel relaxed and your mind has cleared.

BELOW *Place a large crystal in front of you and focus on it for a few moments.*

Sight Focus

The nature of clear quartz makes it an ideal tool for centering and focusing. To get the best results, use a large, self-standing clear quartz crystal or a shaped stone such as an egg or sphere. Place the crystal at a comfortable distance from you so your eyes can rest without straining as you gaze into the center of the quartz crystal. After a few moments, gently close your eyes and rest. If there is still some agitation, repeat the process.

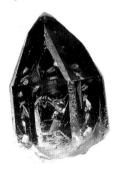

CLEAR QUARTZ

TAPPING IN

Tapping in brings into balance all the major energy meridians of the body for about 20 minutes. It is also one of the simplest and most effective techniques for making sure that a stable, centered energy is kept in place. The following are a couple of variations:

• The simplest procedure is a firm, light tapping with the fingertips on the area of the upper chest just below where the collarbone (clavicle) meets the breast bone (sternum). This is the approximate placement of the thymus gland, which is important for maintenance of the subtle energy balance in the body. If, while the thymus is being tapped, your other hand is placed palm open, over your navel, the balancing effect tends to last longer.

• Another variation of tapping in is to tap counterclockwise as you are looking down on your chest, in a circle about 3 to 6 inches (7–15 cm) away from the thymus point. Each tap of the fingers should be about 1 inch (2.5 cm) apart. Repeat the circle about 20 times.

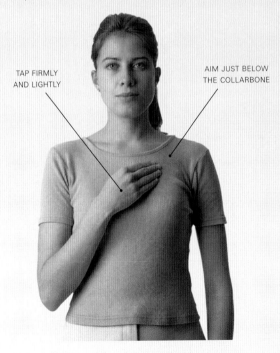

TAP FIRMLY
AND LIGHTLY

AIM JUST BELOW
THE COLLARBONE

• Many important meridian channels pass close to the navel. Tapping around the navel about 3 to 4 inches (7–10 cm) away in a clockwise direction also has a balancing and centering effect.

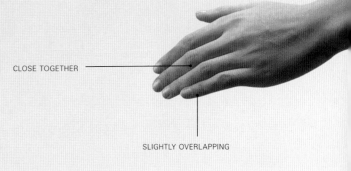

CLOSE TOGETHER

SLIGHTLY OVERLAPPING

• Finally, the thymus and navel tap can be combined in the following way:

1. Hold the fingertips of one hand close together so that they slightly overlap each other.

2. Start off halfway down the center of the chest on the sternum, tapping the fingers onto the rib cage and upper chest at small 1-inch intervals in a counterclockwise circle about 4 to 6 inches (10–15 cm) in diameter.

3. When the starting point is reached again, continue tapping down onto the abdomen, this time creating a clockwise circle around the navel, then returning to the center of the chest. This creates a figure-eight pattern.

4. Repeat this 15 to 20 times.

Tapping in should become an automatic process. The more the body systems become used to existing in a state of harmonious balance, the easier it is to maintain balance and the more apparent it becomes when we lose that balance, thus ensuring that we notice and correct imbalances sooner.

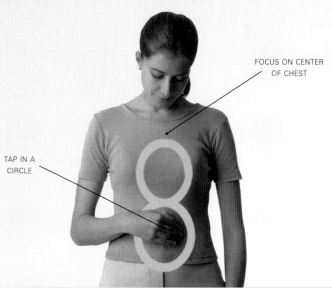

FOCUS ON CENTER OF CHEST

TAP IN A CIRCLE

Voice Focus

Making an open "Ahhh" sound for as long as is comfortable causes the bones and soft tissues of the body to resonate gently and relaxes tension that has accumulated in muscles, particularly the chest, head, and throat. "Ahhh" is the simplest sound that can be made. It doesn't involve any tension in the vocal cords or mouth. Simply breathe out through the mouth and begin the sound. The volume or tone of the sound isn't important. Focus your attention on the quality of the vibration for as long as it can be sustained. Repeat the process as many times as you like. Some people may be familiar with chanting other sounds, such as "Om" or "Aum." This, too, can be a useful centering device, but it requires more vocal control and a little more effort.

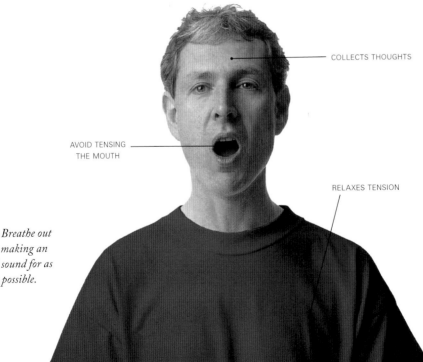

COLLECTS THOUGHTS

AVOID TENSING
THE MOUTH

RELAXES TENSION

RIGHT *Breathe out gently, making an "ahhh" sound for as long as possible.*

Protection and Support

*T*here are times in healing when the healer uncovers issues that are deep-seated, stressful, and difficult to examine. At other times, a problem appears in a patient that closely echoes a difficult personal experience for the healer. This can lead to a confusion of emotions and energy fluctuations in which balance can easily be lost. A simple procedure for checking whether both healer and patient are in need of protection and support can avoid unnecessary stress and can make a crystal healing session much more effective.

A healing session can be likened to a small boat dragging a pond to clear out old debris that has accumuluated on the bottom. When a large object is dislodged and begins to move, it can create numerous ripples and waves that might seem likely to overturn the boat. Protection and support techniques act like a steady hand that stops the violent rocking of the boat.

Protection, in this context, is seen as something that helps a person maintain his or her own energy integrity in a situation in which another strong energy source may interfere with or influence them unduly. If, for example, you are meeting someone who makes you feel threatened, a protection technique would allow you to deal with the situation free from fear. Similarly, if your working environment is full of different electromagnetic frequencies that prove to be tiring or enervating, protection may be appropriate.

While protection offers a means to withstand strong external pressures, support strengthens us internally, neutralizing or removing some of our inner resistance to positive change. Support is like an encouraging word from a guide helping us through tricky terrain.

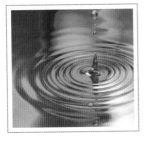

There are many factors in our lives—some seen, some unseen—that can temporarily reduce our effectiveness as a healer. The cause might be something mundane, such as a certain food disagreeing with us, or subtle, such as an astronomical alignment. It is not important to know the exact source of the difficulty, so long as it can be rendered harmless.

After an initial centering and grounding exercise, it is a good idea to carry out a check by dowsing or muscle testing *(see pages 129–137)* in order to learn whether protection and support are needed before any crystal healing work is begun. Should the response be positive, it will then be necessary to find the appropriate solutions.

ABOVE *A crystal healing session can act as a calming influence on the ripples that upset and disturb our lives.*

PROTECTING AND SUPPORT CATEGORIES WITH EXERCISES

BELOW *Eat lots of fresh, unprocessed foods, preferably those produced organically.*

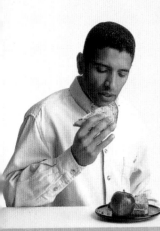

There are many ways of gaining the necessary support and protection. Choose the one that works best for you in a given situation.

GROUNDING: Try exercises such as tree meditation, breathing, centerline breathing, or food for grounding.
NUTRITION: Food for extra energy, vitamin or mineral supplementation, or a drink of water.
EXERCISES: Cook's Hookup, meridian massage, tapping in, or cross-crawl.
SOUND: Mantra, affirmation, toning, chanting or singing, listening to music or sound, or playing music or sound.
SMELL: Essential oils to smell, essential oils to wear, or any other fragrance.
SIGHT: Visualizing a color, looking at a color or combinations of colors, patterns, symbols, mandalas, images (people, animals, a landscape, etc.).
CRYSTALS: Wearing a crystal, carrying a crystal, meditating or attuning to a stone, or looking at a stone.

RIGHT *Fresh fruit and vegetables*

If you are working with another person, carry out the checks, such as dowsing or muscle testing, for both of you. This is particularly important when you know that there are deep underlying stresses or very important issues to be explored during the crystal healing session.

Procedure

Dowse or muscle test using the question: "Do I, or does this person, need protection and support before continuing with this healing procedure?"

• If the answer is no, you can continue as normal, but if the situation becomes emotionally charged during the course of the healing session, ask this question again.

• If the answer is yes, then determine which steps need to be taken.

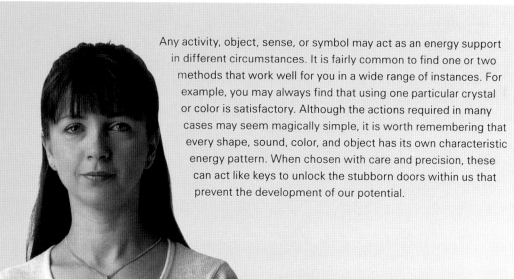

Any activity, object, sense, or symbol may act as an energy support in different circumstances. It is fairly common to find one or two methods that work well for you in a wide range of instances. For example, you may always find that using one particular crystal or color is satisfactory. Although the actions required in many cases may seem magically simple, it is worth remembering that every shape, sound, color, and object has its own characteristic energy pattern. When chosen with care and precision, these can act like keys to unlock the stubborn doors within us that prevent the development of our potential.

LEFT *Wear a carefully selected piece of crystal.*

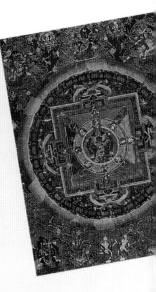

ABOVE *Certain symbols may assist with energy support, like this Buddhist mandala painting.*

Exploring with Crystals

*I*t is a good idea to begin by doing a few simple experiments just to see what differences you notice when using crystals and gemstones. In order to increase your awareness and sensitivity, get used to noticing the differences in how you feel before, during, and after each session. There are two basic methods of placement: one with the points of all the crystals facing inward; the other with all the points facing out from the body. Generally speaking, when the points are outward, they help release imbalances, and when pointing inward, they infuse the body with energy.

BELOW *Begin with a simple crystal placement. Space the crystals out along one side of the body and then along the other.*

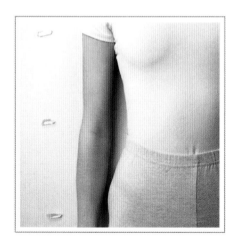

Take time to note down your experiences. This will eventually speed up your growth in confidence and the ability to use your intuition.

Analyzing How You Feel

1. Lie down comfortably for about ten minutes. After this time, note how your body feels, what you were thinking about, and so on.

2. Continue your normal routine for half an hour at least.

3. Then lie down again for about ten minutes. This time use a simple placement of stones, such as one of those suggested on *page 69*, and again record how you feel physically, your thoughts, and so on.

Simple Placements

Take three clear quartz crystals, preferably ones with naturally terminated points, and try each of the following in sequence, spending two or three minutes on each.

1. Place all three crystals, evenly spaced, next to the left side of the body. Start with all the crystals pointing in toward you, and after a minute or so, turn their points away from your body.

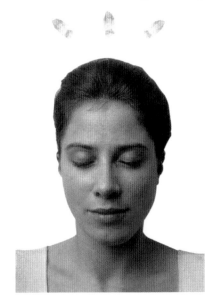

2. Next put all three crystals next to the right side of your body. Again, begin with their points facing inward and then rotate them so they face outward.

3. Now try with all three stones placed around your head—points outward followed by points inward.

4. Follow this by positioning the quartz crystals, points down, below the feet. You will probably notice a difference in sensations within your body. Perhaps your mind will become quieter or busier than usual, or your breathing may alter. Make a note of your experiences, even if it's as vague as feeling comfortable or fidgety. When you have clear results, try with the same stones, but this time place them on your body and see how your experiences differ.

Practical Exercises

We all experience the energy of crystals in different ways. It is much easier to notice a contrasting feeling or sensation than an energy. The following exercises will help identify in which ways a crystal may be acting upon our subtle energy systems and where we might be sensitive to its characteristics.

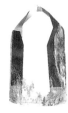

RIGHT *Study the crystal from all angles; imagine it with your eyes shut.*

Remember to cleanse the crystals before beginning *(see pages 29–32).*

With every new stone that you use, it is helpful to repeat the following simple procedures.

1. Hold the stone in both hands close to the solar plexus. As you breathe out, imagine your breath passing over the top of the stone. When you breathe in, see your breath entering the crystal and being drawn into your body. The breath creates a cycle passing from you through the crystal and back into your body. Continue the breathing process for a while and then relax. This is an easy and effective way to integrate a crystal's energy into your own energy.

2. Look closely at the crystal, examining it from as many different angles as possible. Close your eyes, imagine the shapes, and then look again. Then relax and hold the stone in both hands for a minute or two. Make a note of any thoughts or impressions that come to you.

RIGHT *Sketch the crystal, expressing your intuitive feelings about it.*

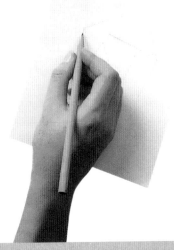

3. Take a good look at the crystal and then quickly draw it large on a sheet of paper. Don't worry about accuracy. Now, imagine and draw how energy seems to move in, through, and around the crystal. Note down any words, thoughts, or images that occur during this time. It is important to relax and be playful here. Suspend any aesthetic or analytical judgments you have if they interfere with your impressions.

4a. Place the crystal on a surface a comfortable distance in front of you. Sit quietly with your eyes closed for a moment.

4b. Open your eyes and look at the crystal before you.

4c. Close your eyes again and sit quietly.

4d. Reach out and pick up the crystal and hold it in both hands for a little while with your eyes closed.

4e. After a minute or two, place the stone back in front of you.

4f. Repeat this picking up and putting down several times and notice any changes in how you feel.

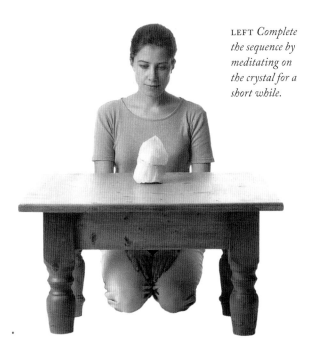

LEFT *Complete the sequence by meditating on the crystal for a short while.*

Simple Healing Layouts

These simple healing layouts are intended to restore the body's natural balance of energies in a general way and to help bring relaxation and a settled, receptive state of mind. If the stones are very small, smooth, or irregular, you may want to tape them in place.

Balancing and Calming

Place a clear quartz point outward at the crown of the head, a small rose quartz in the center of the chest, and a smoky quartz, point downward, close to the base of the spine, between the legs.

Centering and Grounding

This is an excellent way to bring yourself back down to Earth when your thoughts and energies are scattered or when you feel confused. Two smoky quartz crystals are used; one is placed point down at the base of the throat, just above the collarbone; the second stone is placed, point down, at the base of the spine, between the legs.

Feeling Disoriented

This layout is for when you are not quite feeling right but can't figure out why or what to do. Clear quartz is placed at the crown of the head and smoky quartz between the legs, close to the spine. The third stone is placed in the middle of the forehead and can be either a turquoise or a piece of lapis lazuli. If you have both, you might feel more comfortable with one more than the other.

CLEAR QUARTZ

SMOKY QUARTZ

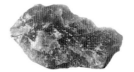

ROSE QUARTZ

BELOW *Clear quartz will clear and balance the mind and upper chakras.*

BELOW *The smoky quartz grounds and focuses you on physical reality.*

BELOW *This layout energizes and balances the chakra energies; it also helps energy flow.*

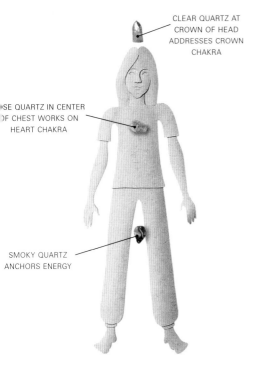

CLEAR QUARTZ AT CROWN OF HEAD ADDRESSES CROWN CHAKRA

SE QUARTZ IN CENTER OF CHEST WORKS ON HEART CHAKRA

SMOKY QUARTZ ANCHORS ENERGY

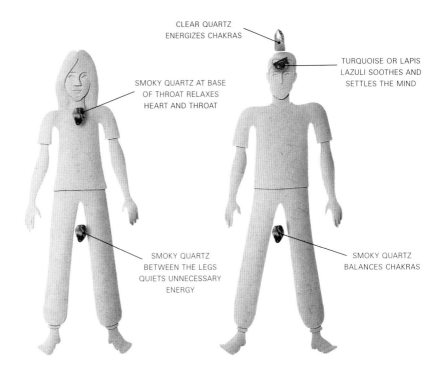

SMOKY QUARTZ AT BASE OF THROAT RELAXES HEART AND THROAT

SMOKY QUARTZ BETWEEN THE LEGS QUIETS UNNECESSARY ENERGY

CLEAR QUARTZ ENERGIZES CHAKRAS

TURQUOISE OR LAPIS LAZULI SOOTHES AND SETTLES THE MIND

SMOKY QUARTZ BALANCES CHAKRAS

ENERGIZING CRYSTALS

RECHARGING BODY AND SPIRIT

Place a quartz crystal on a pulse point or by using several crystals on different pulses. If you are using a single quartz, hold its largest facet gently to the skin. Imagine drawing the sun's rays into your body through the crystal. Doing this in direct sunlight enhances the process.

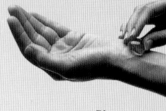

CRYSTALS AND BREATHING

1. Inhale to bring energy into your aura.

2. Hold your breath for three to six seconds and focus your awareness into a crystal in your hand.

3. With a forceful, rapid breathing out, the accumulated energy is projected out through the top of the crystal with intensified force.

4. Point to a specific area that needs healing and use several cycles of the sequence.

ABOVE *Place crystals on both wrists to regulate body energies.*

BELOW *Hold the stone in both hands and draw energy through it.*

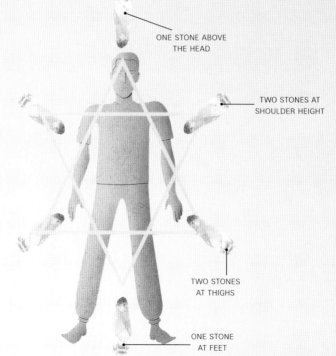

ONE STONE ABOVE THE HEAD

TWO STONES AT SHOULDER HEIGHT

RIGHT *Stones on the body can be held in place by tape.*

TWO STONES AT THIGHS

ONE STONE AT FEET

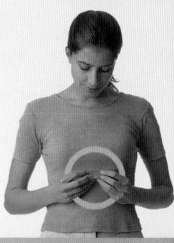

The Seal of Solomon

Also called the Star of David, this layout uses six quartz crystals and forms a six-pointed star. As a healing layout, it is effective and versatile in a wide range of situations.

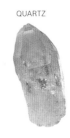

QUARTZ

Begin by placing the stones, points outward, to release any imbalances and tensions. After three or four minutes, reverse the crystals to recharge your energy fields. Be aware of how you feel during this process. If you feel uncomfortable, try changing the direction of the crystals. It is fairly common to find that the charging process needs less time than the cleansing.

The Seal of Solomon can also be used on and around smaller parts of the body to help reduce pain or to give some extra healing energy. Tape stones onto the body. To enhance or direct the healing, put a stone in the center of the star. For example, copper, malachite, or turquoise can reduce swelling; rose quartz or carnelian will calm and heal.

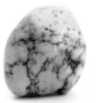
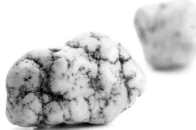

ABOVE *To promote healing, put a stone like turquoise in the center of the star. Turquoise reduces swelling.*

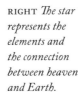
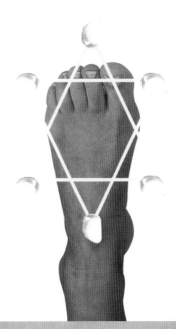

RIGHT *The star represents the elements and the connection between heaven and Earth.*

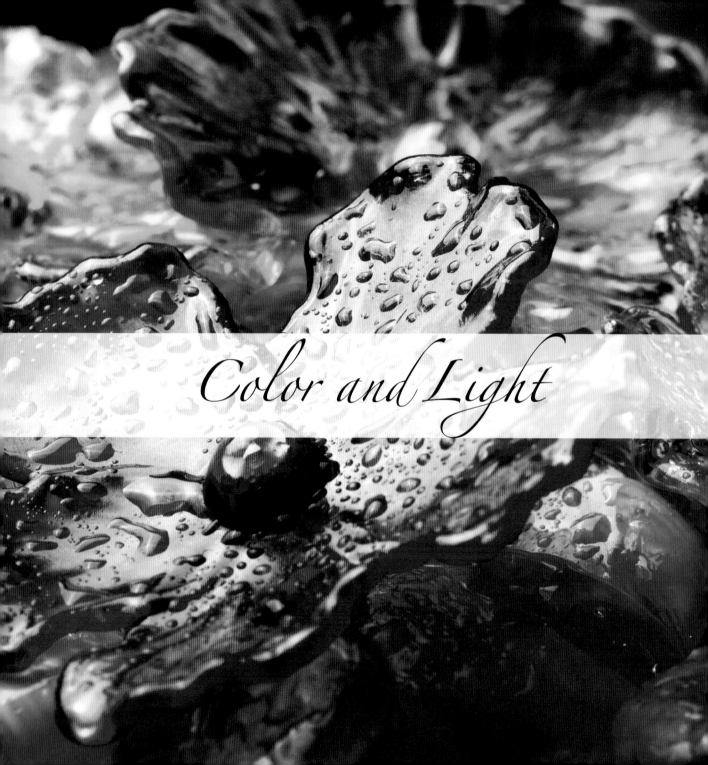

Color and Light

Mineral Colors

The coloration of a crystal results from how it interacts with light, and this is dependent upon the atomic structure of the mineral. There are two main types of mineral colors. Ideochromatic minerals are those, such as copper or chromium, whose chemical composition directly affects their color. Allochromatic minerals, on the other hand, are colored by small amounts of impurities, usually no more than a few atoms of some other element, that create anomalies within the crystal lattice.

In opaque stones the colors we see are those frequencies of light that are not absorbed into the crystal lattice. Where a stone absorbs all frequencies of light, it appears black. White stones reflect the full color spectrum and absorb no light.

With a crystal that is transparent or translucent, light rays enter the crystal structure and are actually slowed down and bent or refracted from their paths by the arrangement of atoms. Depending on how the atoms modify the photons of light, the crystal will shift a full sunlight spectrum toward the slower frequencies, thus appearing red, or toward the faster frequencies of blue and violet. In allochromatic stones, the minute anomalies in the crystal structure carry different energy charges that capture proton particles and form centers of coloration.

When a crystal's color changes according to the angle at which it is viewed, this process is known as pleochromism. The internal structures and symmetry of the mineral break up separate rays of light in different ways,

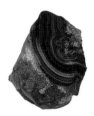

ABOVE
Malachite is an ideochromatic stone, once ground to make a bright green dye.

depending on where the light enters the crystal. Diffraction is where the light becomes polarized, shifting speed and frequency, and emerges from the crystals at different angles.

Color plays a very important role in the process of crystal healing. The characteristic energy vibration or light frequency of each part of the color spectrum affects us at every level—physical, emotional, mental, and spiritual. Learning the key processes and states that each color promotes within us can become a useful foundation both for identifying the general healing effects of a gemstone and for assessing imbalances and their possible roots.

REFRACTION AND DIFFRACTION

When a ray of light passes through a crystal, it is either refracted (bent) or diffracted (diffused) by the arrangement of atoms within the crystal. The color of a crystal depends on whether the light-absorbing atoms shift the light toward the shorter (violet/blue), medium (yellow/green), or longer (orange/red) wavelengths of the light spectrum. White stones reflect the full spectrum, whereas black ones absorb it.

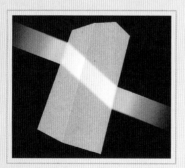

ABOVE *Refraction is when a ray of light is bent as it enters and leaves the crystal.*

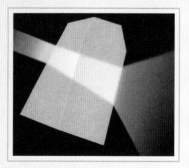

ABOVE *Diffraction is when light is bent off course in various directions.*

Red

*R*ed is associated with heat and dynamism, practical survival drives, lust, energy, and passion. At the physical level, red is associated with activity in general, such as energy and survival. The ability to succeed, skill in the manipulation of physical things, being down-to-earth and businesslike are all manifestations of red energy.

Red is the primary color of the base chakra, or energy center, that connects us to the Earth and to our physical reality. The physical relationship with the color red connects us with the legs, feet, hips, and base of spine. Red is, of course, associated with the circulation system and blood and, on a mineral level, with the iron content of blood.

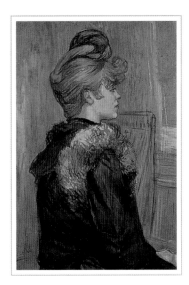

LEFT *Red energy is always directed toward practical creative expression.*

Enthusiasm and drive require red energy. The dynamic, explosive qualities of red energy mean that when it is suppressed or blocked, it can become violent when it finally escapes. The best way to balance red energy is to allow it to flow. Red is the color that is associated with pain, swelling, and inflammation, all heat sensations. Lust for life, a strong sexual drive (libido) and a positive sense of the physical self are also characteristic qualities.

On a mental level, red energy manifests itself as assertiveness and self-confidence and, when out of balance, aggression and arrogance. Red energy is always needed at the beginning of any creative venture. Being grounded, focused, realistic, and in contact with the Earth as well as with the physical body shows a balance of red within an individual.

In its essence, red energy is the passion to be. It is our strength and zest for life. There are many red stones, including garnet, ruby, spinel, zircon, jasper, iron, red quartz, red tourmaline, hematite, and granite.

LEFT *Red stones, like garnets and rubies, are needed before you begin any creative venture.*

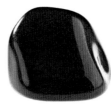

JASPER

GRANITE

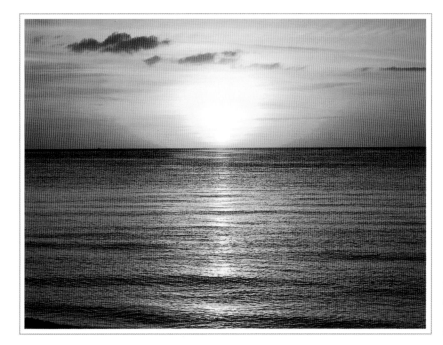

LEFT *Red light energizes many chemical reactions.*

ENERGY IMBALANCES

Indications of a lack of red energy include:

• Cold, inactive, congested conditions.

• Difficulty with physical movement, coordination, or circulation problems.

• Inability to sustain energy levels, physical weakness, and exhaustion.

• Being emotionally and mentally unable to experience life as it is, lacking in drive and enthusiasm, lethargic, uncomfortable with physical activity.

• Feelings of vulnerability and alienation, inability to maintain personal boundaries, easily drained by company.

An excess of red energy might manifest as: hyperactivity, inflammation, physical tension, inability to relax, anger, fear, mental and emotional confusion, rapid mood swings, impatience, fidgeting, intolerance, exasperation, violent outbursts, and exhaustion through continually overextending one's abilities and energy reserves.

Orange

CARNELIAN

*O*range is the energy of red modified by yellow. It takes the raw power of red and channels it in those directions where it is most needed. Red is like the power of a burst dam, while orange is the channel through which that force of water can be harnessed for the benefit of all. Any injury, shock, or trauma, whether life-threatening or transitory, whether physical, emotional, or mental, whether in the distant past or the present, can be dissolved and healed with the help of orange.

Orange vibration stimulates or encourages creativity on all levels for the same reasons that it is effective in healing—because it helps remove any blockage in the way of growth. Orange energy appears in the world as all forms of creative endeavor, including art, music, and healing. It is related to the energy and functions of the second sacral chakra.

The organs within the lower abdomen, especially the large intestine and the reproductive organs, as well as the kidneys higher in the abdominal cavity, all carry out orange-type activities. The kidneys and large intestine are primarily concerned with detoxification and elimination of waste or excess material from the body. These cleansing processes are essential if a buildup of toxins is to be avoided.

Orange at the emotional level works positively with creativity and negatively with stress. With the cleansing and correcting of subtle energy bodies, healing on the physical level speeds up considerably. Because there are fewer disturbances in the flow of energy, conscious awareness can become broader

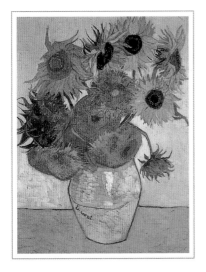

and more receptive. This leads to a clearer understanding at the intuitive levels and to a flowering of wisdom.

Orange stones include tiger's eye, citrine quartz, copper, sun stone, topaz, orange calcite, carnelian, amber, agate, and some garnets. As detoxifiers, Herkimer diamond and selenite also have orange characteristics.

LEFT *Orange energy encourages creativity in all its aspects, inspiring us to continually expand our minds.*

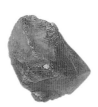

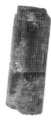

AMBER   ORANGE CALCITE   TOPAZ   COPPER

ENERGY IMBALANCES

A lack of orange energy might manifest itself as:

- Physical rigidity.

- Restricted feelings.

- Digestive disorders.

- Lack of focus.

- Lack of vitality.

- Being stuck in the past, holding onto memories.

The nature of the orange vibration means that it is unusual to find a buildup of excess energy.

Yellow

AGATE

*Y*ellow is the color of the sun, and like the sun, yellow energy tends to make us feel happy and in harmony with our surroundings. At a physical level, the yellow vibration is associated with the solar plexus chakra and with the upper abdomen. The digestive system identifies and selects useful energy sources from the food that we eat and absorbs and assimilates nutrients. The yellow energy expresses intelligence and clarity. A key function of the yellow vibration is the ability to recognize what is useful and what is harmful. Many other physical systems, such as the immune system, rely on the yellow vibration. Recognition of significant danger, such as harmful organisms, is required.

BELOW *Like all colors, the exact shade of yellow will alter our response. A warm golden yellow elicits comfort and happiness, while lemon yellow is mentally stimulating.*

The skin and the nervous system are also yellow in function. Both transmit information and help define where and what we are in relation to our surroundings. Yellow energy in the world expresses itself as all those organizations and activities that use information, organize, and lay down rules and regulations to maintain order. Law, education, and information technology all function by defining and creating boundaries. Emotionally, yellow energy positively translates as feelings of joy, happiness, and contentment. Negatively, it becomes fear, worry, anxiety, and panic. The source of these negative emotions is usually confusion and lack of knowledge. We panic because we lack the right information to know what to do next. Once there is a clear idea of what we can do, confusion vanishes and choices

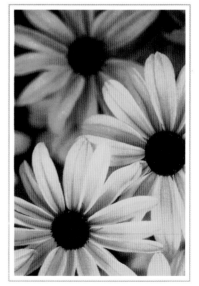

become clear. Yellow emotional states are thus a response to our mental state. Where yellow energy is strong, there is clear knowledge of who one is and how to interact with the world.

Yellow stones are not the most common of minerals, though many do sometimes display this color. Iron pyrites (fool's gold), gold, amber, light citrine quartz, lemon quartz, yellow sapphire, yellow jasper, agate, heliodor (yellow beryl), and fluorite are all in the yellow family.

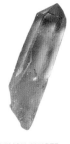

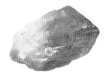

LEMON QUARTZ   HELIODOR   CITRINE

ENERGY IMBALANCES

Physical imbalances of yellow energy might manifest as:

• Stress-related ailments, such as indigestion, insomnia, panic attacks, headaches, muscle tension.

• Skin complaints, such as eczema and psoriasis.

• Nervous disorders.

• Allergic reactions, food intolerance, or arthritis.

• Tension, worry, and confusion.

An excess of yellow mental energy could be exhibited as:

• Overanalytical, fussy behavior.

• Narrow conceptual categorizations, prejudices, and lack of tolerance.

Green

PERIDOT

*G*reen is the primary color of vegetation and has associations with life, growth, and the world of nature. Green is the color of harmonious balance, a calming, restful energy that is linked with the central chakra, the heart.

Physically, green is associated with the heart, lungs, diaphragm, and the arms and hands. The functions of respiration, growth, and the ability to change and adapt are closely linked with this color.

Green is associated with our personal space and a sense of freedom with the ability, or lack of ability, to express ourselves from the heart.

The basis of green energy is the need to grow, expand, and increase our influence and power. It is able to achieve this only by balancing polarities. At a physical level, green links all the systems and organs of the body that maintain balance. At an emotional level, green reflects the balance within the heart. Loving, caring, and sharing are the expansive, inclusive qualities of this color, expanding the self by establishing relationships with others. Relationships also require balance and an interplay of opposites such as freedom and restraint, independence and dependence, sharing and privacy.

Mentally, green energy gives structure to our existence. Routine and discipline may seem to be restrictions to some, but they do create a framework within which freedom can be experienced in a more positive way. Green energy expands from the level of the heart where something is felt to be true. This level of intuitive activity draws on what has gone before it, yet adds a new dimension of personal

BELOW *Green is the color of the vibrant world of nature and our need to experience it.*

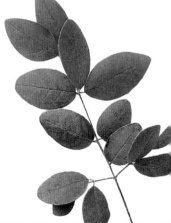

ENERGY IMBALANCES

Green imbalances comprise anything that intrudes into or restricts personal boundaries and equilibrium, including:

• Invasive illness.

• Abnormal growths.

• Lack of control at any level.

• Sense of claustrophobia, being trapped, unfulfilled, restricted, dominated.

• A need to be in control or to be controlled.

• Lack of self-discipline.

• Confusion as to who one is and what direction should be taken and isolation.

BELOW *Green energy keeps us calm and balanced, while also encouraging spiritual growth.*

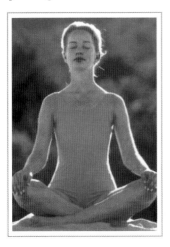

CALCITE

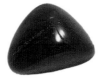

AVENTURINE

DIOPTASE

interpretation. Expansion of knowledge, invention, and innovation are all green mental qualities.

Spiritually, the green vibration relates to all aspects of personal growth and the ability to discern and travel our own personal road.

Green stones include aventurine, jade, peridot, malachite, tourmaline, calcite, moss agate, emerald, garnet, and dioptase.

Blue and Indigo

LAPIS LAZULI

*L*ike its complementary color orange, blue is about flow and communication on all levels, from the interstellar to the cellular. Whenever there is a buildup of tension, a sensation of friction or frustration, or a blocking of energies, blue light will restore the flow. Blue light has been used for years in orthodox medicine as a quick way to reduce inflammation and other hot conditions, such as burns and arthritic pain. Blue is the antidote to any overconcentration of energy and is the opposite to red light in this respect.

Physically, the color blue connects with the throat and brow chakras. It covers the neck, throat, face, ears, eyes, nose, mouth, and forehead. All forms of communication, expression, and learning are blue in quality.

At an emotional level, the color blue can create a flow that helps understanding, empathy, appreciation, and acceptance. It is a color that can reduce the irritation we feel when something jars against our own preferences or beliefs. By increasing our ability to communicate with others and express ourselves effectively, the blue energy can prevent the buildup of friction that would otherwise develop into a red condition of anger.

Self-expression and communication are basic human requirements. We need to see a response from others; we need some form of acknowledgment. The punishment of ignoring and excluding someone from the personal community is emotionally and psychologically damaging. When there is an excess of blue energy, its coolness can become all-enveloping. Emotional detachment and mental aloofness are the result.

CELESTITE

ENERGY IMBALANCES

Indicators of blue imbalances are:

• Throat problems, laryngitis, sore throats, and tonsillitis (these all suggest difficulties within the sphere of personal communication, either at an everyday level or sometimes simply the need to become involved in some artistic activity).

• Blocks to creativity and inspiration.

• Cold, congested states show and excess of blue.

Extreme agitated states can be helped with blue initially, although the calming qualities of green are more suitable in the long term.

Blue is not a color to use in cases of depression, nor should it be used for extended periods without the balancing effect of more activating colors.

Blue is a color that can increase our ability to contact the deep areas of the mind where inspiration and the imagination reside. It also allows intuition to flourish, and at the same time its cool quality means that information coming from the finer levels of the mind can be looked at and assessed clearly without interference from any inappropriate responses. Seeing clearly, perceiving, and understanding sum up the effects of blue energy.

Blue stones and crystals range from the light blue of celestite, blue topaz, aquamarine, blue lace agate, and blue calcite to the dark blues of lapis lazuli, blue quartz, indicolite or blue tourmaline, kyanite, sapphire, and azurite.

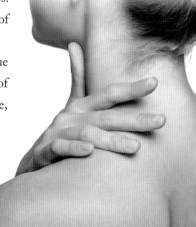

BELOW *Throat problems, such as laryngitis or tonsillitis, are indicators of blue energy imbalances.*

Violet

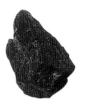

SUGILITE

*T*he key to understanding violet energy is in the combination of its constituent colors blue and red. The energy of violet is a synthesis of the hot, activating, dynamic, manifesting quality of red with the cooling, sedating, pacifying, dematerializing quality of blue. The tones of violet are thus a spiritualization of matter and an energizing of spirit—a union of apparent opposites.

Physically, the violet vibration relates to the crown chakra and the head generally, but specifically the cranium or the skull. It also connects the functions of the brain to the pituitary and pineal glands.

Within the physical body, violet energy works to create coordination and integration between the physical systems. Physical coordination problems and learning difficulties in children often arise from an imbalance between the left and right hemispheres of the brain.

The tendency to switch off, or not recognize, what is going on at some level is a very violet characteristic of imbalance on any level.

Violet energy provides the flow of information via the blue qualities, together with the activating energy of the life force via the red. Together, they serve as a switch to turn on those mechanisms that will help the body recognize and deal with situations of imbalance and illness. This makes violet one of the most useful, generally applicable, healing energies in crystal work.

Violet energy at an emotional level tends to foster understanding and sympathy for others, and at a mental level opens the awareness to imagination and inspiration. Violet encourages all aspects of artistic expression and

ENERGY IMBALANCES

Violet imbalance can become extreme, expressing itself as:

• An exaggerated need to sacrifice for others, which often disguises guilt or poor self-worth.

• A tendency to live in a world of illusory value judgments or to escape into fantasy and daydreaming.

• Delusional states and reinterpretation of reality based on personal fanaticism.

The following can be helped by violet energy:

• Headaches.

• Problems with eyes and ears.

• Deep-seated glandular imbalances and other chronic imbalances of the whole system.

• Lack of focus mentally and spiritually, inability to concentrate, failure to understand what is happening in life or to change.

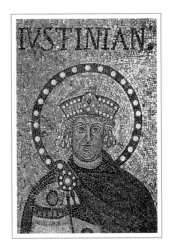

ABOVE *Related to the crown chakra, violet is associated with conscious awareness and reflective thinking.*

practical problem solving. The expansive nature of the vibration also helps enter and maintain meditative states.

Violet and purple stones are not frequently found and can be rare and expensive. The most common and most broadly effective is amethyst quartz. Others include fluorite, sugilite, charoite, tanzanite, iolite or water sapphire, lepidolite, and kunzite.

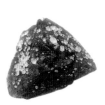

FLUORITE

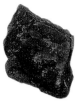

IOLITE

CHAROITE

Pink and Turquoise

RHODOCROSITE

*P*ink is a combination of white and red and so tends to be dynamic, expressing the energy and activation of red with the all-encompassing, cleansing qualities of white. Jealousies, aggression, and misunderstandings all fade away when illuminated by the pink vibration. Whenever there is a violent or negative situation, the use of pink light for short periods of time quickly re-establishes calm.

Visualizing a pale or pure pink light emanating from one's heart dispels negativity, and projecting pink around or at someone who is aggressive toward you or who is annoying you, will help calm the situation before it gets out of hand.

In crystal therapy, pink is found with green at the heart center, where it is used to help release emotional stress. All issues to do with self-image can be greatly helped by pink light. Pink energy increases levels of tolerance

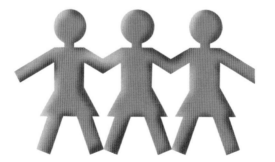

LEFT *Pink is a unifier, reinforcing the link that all things have to each other and quickly neutralizing all false divisions.*

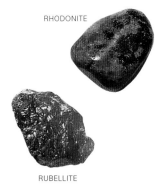

RHODONITE

RUBELLITE

and sympathy and the effectiveness of healing. It works well as first-aid and in the release of long-term trauma.

Pink-colored stones include rose quartz, rubellite (pink tourmaline), rhodonite, rhodocrosite, kunzite, cherry opal, coral, and thulite.

TURQUOISE

Turquoise comes in a variety of shades between green and blue. The heart center, represented by green energy, is linked together with the throat chakra, the light blue energy, indicating that turquoise helps articulate and express the true wishes of the heart. Expression of the uniqueness of each individual is a powerful and essential part of everyone's life. Turquoise reaffirms our sense of value and purpose and significantly increases the life energy available to each of us. Consider using turquoise in any situation where stress and illness are clearly draining the individual. Turquoise-colored stones include aquamarine, turquoise, chrysocolla, larimar, gem silica, and amazonite.

CHRYSOCOLLA

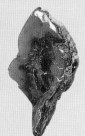

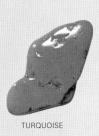

TURQUOISE

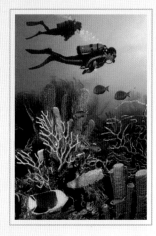

ABOVE *The light blue energy of turquoise is the means by which our desire for growth is communicated.*

White

MOONSTONE

*W*hite is the union of all colors, so essentially it has the potential to become any color. White is the vibration of pure potential. Everything exists within it and anything might manifest from it, yet white itself displays no characteristics. In practical terms, white will supply whatever energy is needed.

White light is the complete, unseparated spectrum and reflects all energies out from itself. When combined with another color, white will amplify and augment that color. When talking about crystals and color, white includes those crystals that are clear, which allow light to pass through them unaltered. Stones that appear white in color are reflecting all frequencies of light from their surfaces.

White has no clear connection to the physical body, although it is often associated with the area just above the top of the head at or above the crown chakra. At an emotional level, white feels cold and undefined. Since it cannot absorb anything, it remains somewhat remote and inviolable, hence its ties to purity. The purification that white light brings is rapid and unequivocal, and as such it can be a harsh experience. But if the

BELOW *In Native American tradition, white is assigned to the north, from where comes snow and ice.*

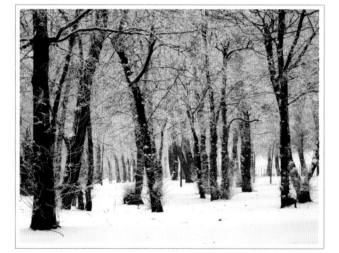

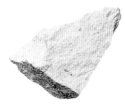

CHALK

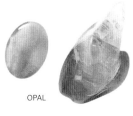

OPAL

more temperate color of orange doesn't free up blockages, then white light might be successful.

With white light, all shadows and distinctions dissolve. It can be utterly cleansing, stripping away all masks and pretensions and destroying everything that is not part of your true nature, so it should always be used with caution. White is the brand-new start, the blank page. The projection of emptiness can seem remote and unsympathetic until the time comes when it is absolutely necessary to use its powerful frequency.

Clear stones that reflect the purifying force of white light are clear quartz, Herkimer diamond, diamond, Iceland spa (a variety of calcite), and gypsum, selenite, and apophyllite.

White stones include milky quartz, moonstone, opal, and chalk.

ICELAND SPA

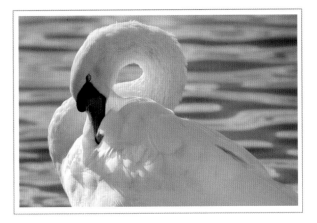

ABOVE *Culturally, white has diverse meanings: in the modern West, white relates to cleanliness, purity, and the spirit, while in China white is the color of death.*

Black

OBSIDIAN

*B*lack contains all colors within itself and absorbs all the energies into itself so that no light at all can be seen. A black hole exists because its immense gravity draws all matter, time, and light into itself. Black, in the same way, is the ultimate expression of gravity, pulling everything inward to experience its core, central nature.

Blackness as an experience can be frightening because of its lack of definition. Anything or everything may be out there in the dark. But everything may include all the good, beneficial experiences as well as terrors and fears. In this way, the lesson of black is the same as white. It contains within itself all potential, but where white will create the energy for a rapid, immediate change of state, black will allow a rest period, a dormancy within which growth and change can begin to take shape.

All aspects of the hidden—the concealed factors, the subconscious and unconscious, and everything that is not in the present moment of conscious awareness—can be represented by the color black.

Black can be a good grounding color because it contacts the deepest, most solid foundations of any situation. Black can also be the means by which the underlying, hidden factors and emotions can be brought to the surface and examined.

As an energy of meditation, the color black can be extremely useful. It creates a restful and tranquil silence in which it is possible to explore deep levels.

Black is also a very protective color, not only because it hides but also because it absorbs all energy, no matter what the source. The combination of black and white can produce an extremely powerful blending of both protective and cleansing qualities.

Black stones include schorl or black tourmaline, smoky quartz, obsidian, jet, and onyx.

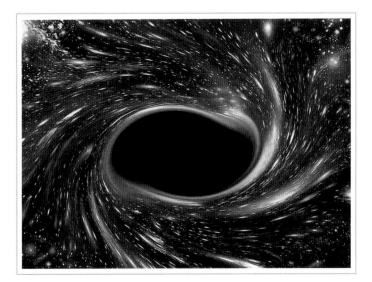

LEFT *The rainbow swirl of colors is pulled in and absorbed by a black hole in deep space. Black indicates rest and dormancy.*

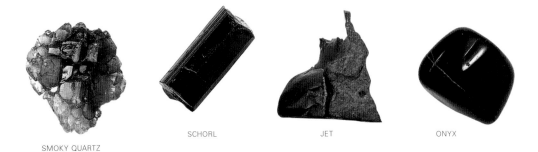

SMOKY QUARTZ
ELESTIAL

SCHORL

JET

ONYX

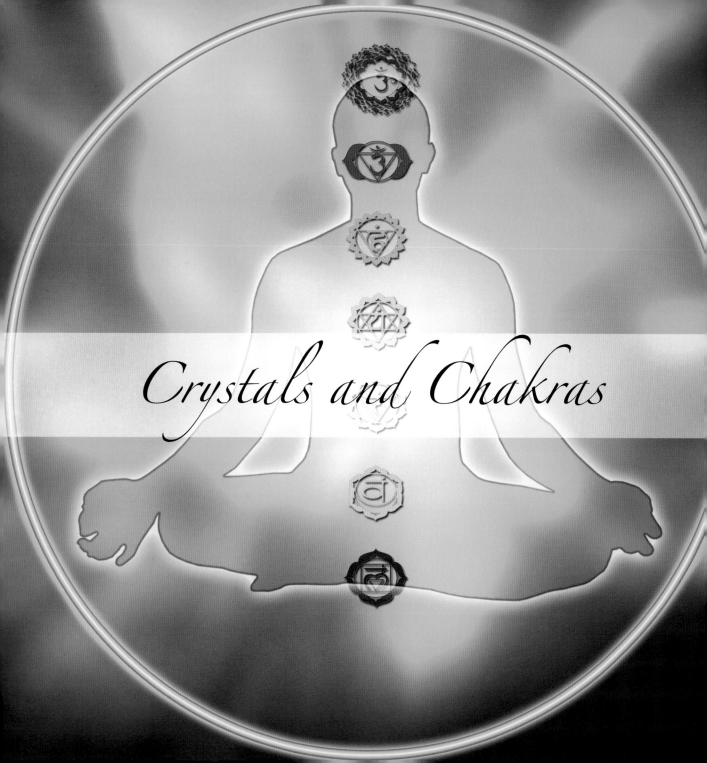

Crystals and Chakras

The Chakra System

Ancient texts from northern India describe a system of subtle channels that run through the body. Arising from the central channel, along the spinal cord, are seven main energy centers, called chakras. The seven main chakras are located close to concentrations of nerves and lymphatic tissues. Aligned, too, are some of the main endocrine glands in the physical body. Although there is no evidence of a direct connection between the body's different systems, it may help explain why the placement of crystals around those areas has such a noticeable effect.

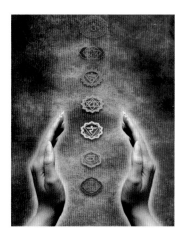

Each chakra can be visualized as a complex meeting point of many different streams of energy. A chakra is the location where a multitude of different influences interact with the human being. Each chakra, although physically separated along the spine, has complex interactions with every other center so that every change in one will affect the functioning of the others. The chakras transmit life-sustaining energy into the body, from our environment and also from multidimensional and universal sources. This energy is distributed into the rest of the body from each chakra point through a number of very subtle channels or nerves known as "nadis."

ABOVE *The seven main chakras.*

The chakras can be seen as a series of elevators that have particular activities, which can move energy through every level of our bodies from the most subtle, spiritual substance down to the physical cells and organs. When they are working in a coherent and orderly way, balance is maintained throughout the whole human being.

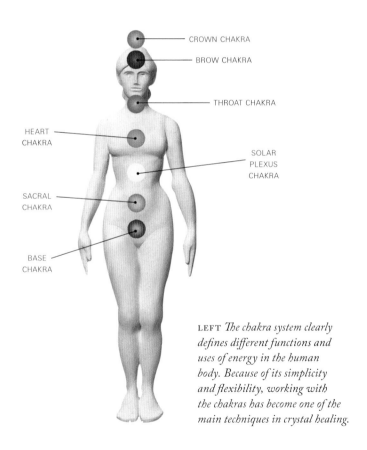

CROWN CHAKRA

BROW CHAKRA

THROAT CHAKRA

HEART
CHAKRA

SOLAR
PLEXUS
CHAKRA

SACRAL
CHAKRA

BASE
CHAKRA

LEFT *The chakra system clearly defines different functions and uses of energy in the human body. Because of its simplicity and flexibility, working with the chakras has become one of the main techniques in crystal healing.*

If, however, over time, a chakra accumulates stress, it will become less able to absorb and process the appropriate energy. This, in turn, will upset the activity of the other chakras. Eventually, if not corrected, this may contribute to physical illness or mental and emotional upset.

In the original Indian descriptions of their functions, the chakras were intended to direct the aspirant to meditations that would help them achieve spiritual growth and so they emphasized the qualities of the chakras above the heart center. But in order to function properly in the everyday world of work, relationships, and practical living, it is essential that all seven main chakras are given equal attention. Perhaps the original writers assumed that in the well-balanced, communal society of the time, the three lower chakras—base, sacral, and solar plexus—were already fully functioning and required little clearing.

The goal of a chakra balance in crystal healing should be to return each chakra to its optimal working state in harmonious relationship with the other energy systems. There is always a certain degree of natural flexibility in each system to take account of individual life patterns and differing requirements, and this awareness in a crystal healer will help achieve maximum benefit from a healing session.

LEFT *In India, chakras were intended to direct participants to meditation that would help them achieve spiritual growth.*

The Base Chakra

The first chakra, called the base, is found at the lower end of the spine. For crystal work, the whole area around the base of the spine can be used for stone placements, especially the groin points (where the legs meet the torso) and between the legs from the knees to the thighs.

The base chakra is the foundation upon which every other body system relies for stability. It is the primary source of usable energy, drawn upon in times of danger to supply energy and physical solutions to life-threatening problems.

The base chakra is vital if we are to keep a grip on reality. A block or stress within this chakra can lead to feelings of unreality, isolation, or an inability to cope. There may be a sense of pointlessness and an inability to achieve goals.

Centering and grounding are key attributes of the base chakra, establishing us firmly within our physical system, alerting us to the world around us, and protecting our energies from depletion. At a physical level, the base chakra can improve circulation of the blood. Problems with the feet and legs, movement, and coordination indicate a need to work with this center. Working with the base chakra, together with the sacral chakra, can help arthritis and lower gastrointestinal disorders.

This chakra's ability to ground excess energy as well as to assimilate it means that when it is stimulated by appropriate crystal placements, it can help release stress, creating a greater ability to relax physically, to let go of worries, and to focus on the enjoyment of the present moment.

LEFT *The base chakra.*

BASE CHAKRA LAYOUT

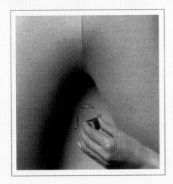

LEFT *To boost the base chakra, place the stones next to, or on, the body.*

There are many ways to place crystals that will strengthen the activities of the base chakra. Here is a layout that can support and enhance the natural functioning of this center. It is designed to help the release of stress and encourage healing. The position of the stones is not important; some can be on the body, others next to it. Stones can be close together in a small area or spread out to cover the whole area of the hips and base of the spine. Place four clear quartz crystals diagonally in a square, pointing outward. Between these stones put four dark tourmalines, also with points outward if they have any. In the center place a red, brown, or black stone.

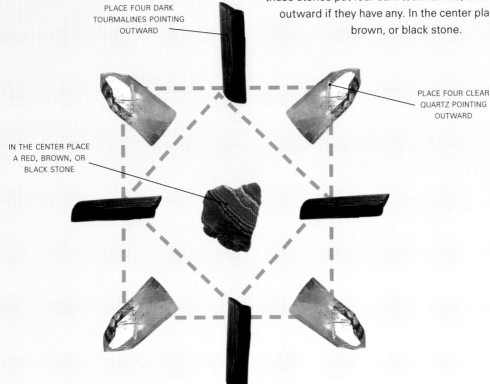

PLACE FOUR DARK TOURMALINES POINTING OUTWARD

PLACE FOUR CLEAR QUARTZ POINTING OUTWARD

IN THE CENTER PLACE A RED, BROWN, OR BLACK STONE

Sacral Chakra

The second chakra is associated with the qualities of movement and flow of energy. It is usually known as the sacral, or sexual, chakra and is placed near the sacrum on the spine. On the front of the body, it is on the lower abdomen between the navel and the pubic bone at the center of the pelvis. Essentially, the purpose of this center is to allow us to explore and enjoy our existence, and to develop emotions and attachments.

This chakra is often under stress from its negative characteristics of rigidity and restriction. The rigidity can be at a physical level with tension and pain in the lower back, digestive problems of the lower intestine, or bladder or kidney trouble. It may manifest as sexual tension, either emotionally triggered or with physical symptoms that can cause impotence or frigidity, and as menstrual pain and irregular periods. Using crystal healing to balance the sacral chakra energies can help by releasing these built-up toxins.

The sacral chakra is also where our deep emotional responses are registered. Suppressed emotions may get locked in our muscle structures and subtle energy systems. They can manifest as anxiety, anger, frustration, and aggression, depriving us of the enjoyment of playfulness and creativity. Tension and fear can alienate us from ourselves and from our surroundings. Blocked energy disrupts normal function and can lead to illness. Working on the sacral chakra can help us keep the spontaneity in our lives. It will release blocks, stress, and trauma and detoxify the whole system.

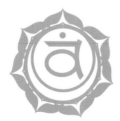

LEFT *The sacral chakra.*

SACRAL CHAKRA LAYOUT

A layout to stimulate the second chakra can be put on the lower abdomen. A downward-pointing triangle is made using three clear crystals. The crystals can be three clear quartz, rutilated quartz, Herkimer diamond, or even diamond. Below this triangle, make an arc of a further three stones, again all of the same kind, choosing from moonstone, rose quartz, lapis lazuli, aquamarine, sugilite, amethyst, charoite, or blue quartz. The stones you decide to use will depend upon what is available and most appropriate for the individual.

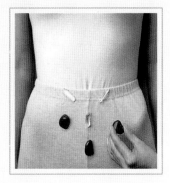

LEFT *Working on this area will release blocks, stress, and trauma and detoxify the whole system.*

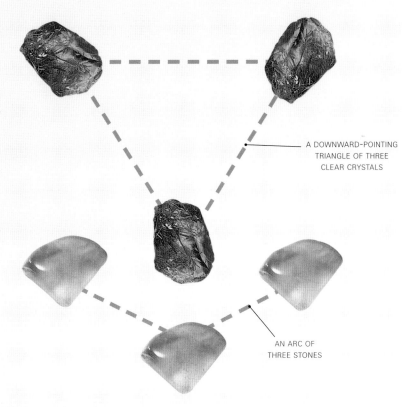

A DOWNWARD-POINTING TRIANGLE OF THREE CLEAR CRYSTALS

AN ARC OF THREE STONES

Solar Plexus Chakra

The third, or solar plexus, chakra motivates us to bring about change. This fiery chakra deals with our use of energy and ability to transform it from a raw state into usable forms. The solar plexus chakra is an organizing control center that gives us the will and ability to mold our lives in a powerful, effective way. It integrates us actively into the world. Optimism, self-confidence, spontaneity, flexibility, a sense of humor, joy, and laughter are the balanced expression of the solar plexus.

Located between the base of the rib cage and the navel, the solar plexus chakra covers the major areas of digestion, such as the stomach, small intestine, liver, and pancreas, as well as the spleen, one of the most important organs of the immune system, which relies on its ability to recognize what is useful and to identify and destroy harmful organisms. The solar plexus chakra also plays a part in the functioning of the skin and nervous system, both of which depend on communication and identification of outside messages.

Indications that the solar plexus needs support can be overacidity, ulcers, digestive problems, allergies and intolerance, and difficulties with immune system function from constant colds and persistent viral infections. More serious problems may include autoimmune disorders, chronic fatigue, burnout, or hypertension. On an emotional level, look for anxiety, stress, lack of confidence, insecurity, or nervous disorders. Working with the solar plexus chakra can be important for stress reduction and relaxation.

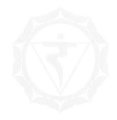

LEFT *The solar plexus chakra.*

SOLAR PLEXUS CHAKRA LAYOUT

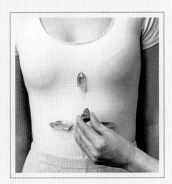

LEFT *When crystals begin to release tension, there may be an increase in deep, full breaths, sighs, or yawning.*

Arrange the following stones on the upper abdomen between the lower edge of the rib cage, near the diaphragm and the navel. Make an upward-pointing triangle of three citrine quartz crystals, with points facing outward. In the center of this triangle, place one of the following: tiger's eye, ruby, garnet, jasper, or iron pyrite. The stone you place here will determine the quality of energy being balanced. For example, the red stones of ruby and garnet will energize, or jasper and pyrites are grounding and aid digestion. Tiger's eye will ground and encourage practical social skills. Surrounding these four stones, make another triangle, this time with three garnets pointing downward.

A DOWNWARD-
POINTING TRIANGLE
USING THREE GARNETS

A CENTRAL CRYSTAL
SUCH AS RUBY WILL
ENERGIZE

AN UPWARD-POINTING
TRIANGLE USING THREE
CITRINE QUARTZ

Heart Chakra

At the center of the chest is the heart chakra. This is the midpoint of the entire chakra system, with three above and three below. Balance and equilibrium are the keys to understanding heart chakra energies. Complete wellness begins and ends with the balance within the heart.

The heart works by alternately contracting and expanding, as it pumps blood around the body. The lungs inhale air by expanding and contracting. Both these systems only work when a balance is maintained. This equilibrium of opposite actions maintains the friction and flow of life energy through the universe.

When the heart chakra is balanced, there is a sense of calm, clearsighted-ness, and tolerance of others. We know where we want to go, and we can hold our own ground as well.

When the heart chakra is out of balance, it is easy to lose our own understanding of our relationship with the world, becoming possessive or obsessive, constantly seeking reassurance, and experiencing self-doubt lack of self-worth. These imbalances can lead to cold, emotionless power-seeking, intolerance, prejudice, and cruelty. On the other hand, there can be an overwhelming sense of personal responsibility for other people's welfare, leading to desperate self-sacrifice and guilt that undermines all sense of self-worth.

The heart chakra is a vital healing location, where the swings of polarized emotions, feelings, hopes, and wishes can be evened out and a positive calm can be restored in which to re-establish a life-supporting relationship with the world.

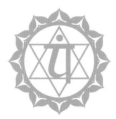

LEFT *The heart chakra.*

HEART CHAKRA LAYOUT

Put a rose quartz at the center of the chest. Make a cross with points outward around this along the axes of the body. The cross can be made with green tourmaline crystals or, alternatively, clear quartz, rose quartz, or another other pink crystal. If tumbled stones are used here, add clear quartz points to direct the energy out and away from the center stone. Midway in the first cross place another of four outward-pointing smoky quartz crystals. This layout balances the heart chakra. Where there is a need to clarify goals or fulfill desires, place a a Herkimer diamond just below the arrangement. A small chakra, the Anandakanda Lotus, is located here, and that helps to access our true nature.

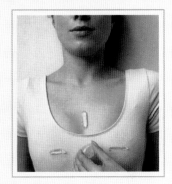

RIGHT *When the heart chakra is fully balanced, the entire chakra system works in harmony.*

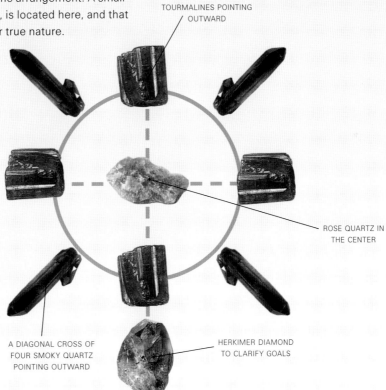

A CROSS USING GREEN TOURMALINES POINTING OUTWARD

ROSE QUARTZ IN THE CENTER

A DIAGONAL CROSS OF FOUR SMOKY QUARTZ POINTING OUTWARD

HERKIMER DIAMOND TO CLARIFY GOALS

Throat Chakra

The throat chakra is found at the base of the throat around the sternal notch, where the collarbone meets the sternum. Physically, this chakra is related to the thyroid and parathyroid glands and to the upper chest, neck, throat, mouth, nose, and ears. The shoulders, arms, and hands can be affected by both the heart and throat chakras.

The throat chakra is concerned with communication—it allows us to transmit our thoughts, ideas, and desires. It is also the means by which we express our creativity.

Sore throats and stiff necks can often be indications that there is a problem with some level of communication. Often something is being held back by force of will that would be better verbalized in some way, or a desire to express individuality is also being stifled.

Without this natural flow of communicated energy traveling out into the world, other sorts of energies also slow down, and there is a danger of stagnation. At the physical level, thyroid activity may be disrupted, leading to states of either lethargy or hyperactivity. Muscle stiffness in the neck, shoulders, and jaw results from a lack of energy flow in those areas. Chronic tension in the jaw can lead to headaches.

On an emotional level, throat chakra problems can lead to an inability to express and feel emotions at a deeper level. This dissociation can lead to withdrawal and isolation or, alternatively, can create a chatterbox who doesn't feel comfortable unless talking, but doesn't communicate any true feeling.

LEFT *The throat chakra.*

THROAT CHAKRA LAYOUT

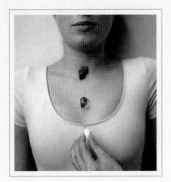

LEFT *The throat chakra is closely connected to the mind and all aspects of education, learning, understanding, and knowledge.*

One way to rebalance the throat chakra is to place a blue stone near the sternal notch. Close beneath this, near the thymus gland, put a turquoise-colored stone. Below this on the breastbone, set a downward-pointing clear quartz crystal. Finally on each side of the uppermost blue stone, place a crystal with double terminations or points at each end. These two crystals can be of any sort so long as they are the same stone. Probably small quartz crystals with natural double terminations will be easiest to find.

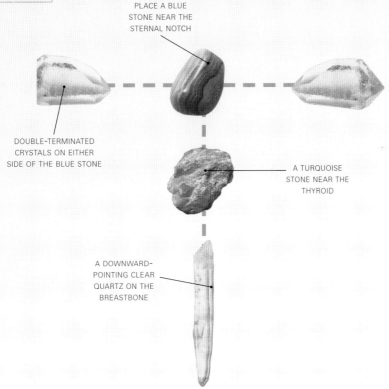

PLACE A BLUE STONE NEAR THE STERNAL NOTCH

DOUBLE-TERMINATED CRYSTALS ON EITHER SIDE OF THE BLUE STONE

A TURQUOISE STONE NEAR THE THYROID

A DOWNWARD-POINTING CLEAR QUARTZ ON THE BREASTBONE

Brow Chakra

The sixth, or brow, chakra is the fabled "third eye." Its primary function is concerned with the understanding and analysis of reality. It differs from the throat chakra in that it has a more passive quality; the brow chakra is inward-looking rather than expressive in its nature.

Physically, it is in the area of the center of the forehead that is sometimes defined as between the eyebrows. The eyes and the conscious workings of the brain are directly related to the brow chakra, whose main function is to make sense of the raw information received from the sense organs. It also works with memory and planning, by receiving and analyzing information from the remembered past and the projected future. The brow chakra is the focus of our personality, for our view of reality is an expression of who we are and how we see ourselves in relation to the universe.

When this chakra loses its balance with the system as a whole, the mind has a tendency to retreat from reality into the self-constructed realms of fantasy and delusion. The brow chakra needs integrated balance and a firm grounded energy if it is to be of real use to us.

With an active but imbalanced brow chakra, it is possible to see visions, receive messages from the subtle senses (like clairvoyance), and be bombarded by intriguing psychic information. But unless there is a balanced and equal emphasis on the energies of the base, sacral, and solar plexus chakras, it is almost impossible to determine what is valid and useful.

LEFT *The brow chakra.*

BROW CHAKRA LAYOUT

The brow chakra is extemely sensitive, so placing an appropriate crystal on the forehead can have a profound balancing effect. A balancing layout for the brow chakra is as follows:

In the center of the forehead place either a Herkimer diamond or lapis lazuli. On each side of it, set a small fluorite crystal of any color. These should be positioned approximately at the center of the eyebrows. Another fluorite goes right above the first central stone. An optional blue or violet fluorite can be added near the top of the head, by the crown.

RIGHT *Crystals can bring out the best qualities of the brow chakra, including an expansive intuition focused sharply by a clear, perceptive mind.*

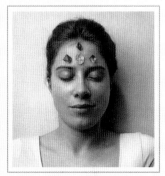

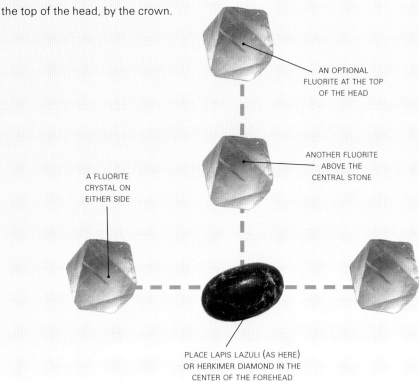

AN OPTIONAL
FLUORITE AT THE TOP
OF THE HEAD

ANOTHER FLUORITE
ABOVE THE
CENTRAL STONE

A FLUORITE
CRYSTAL ON
EITHER SIDE

PLACE LAPIS LAZULI (AS HERE)
OR HERKIMER DIAMOND IN THE
CENTER OF THE FOREHEAD

Crown Chakra

The seventh, or crown, chakra is said to be located a distance of four finger-breadths above the top of the head, although in practical terms the whole area of the crown and above can be used. The crown chakra is our connection to the whole of creation. Aspects of this wholeness are filtered, transformed, and utilized by the rest of the chakra system.

When the crown chakra loses its balance, a shadow is cast over the whole system. There is a feeling that something is not right. Feelings of alienation and depression, and of a weight descending that makes one listless, exhausted, and prone to boredom, all signal a possible crown chakra imbalance.

Physically, apart from its links with the pituitary gland, which it may subtly energize, the crown chakra directly affects the functions of the higher brain, called the cerebrum. A lack of balance between the left and right hemispheres of the brain can cause confusion and coordination difficulties both physically and mentally.

When balanced, the crown chakra increases the ability to understand things in a wider context. This allows the individual to become more intuitive and more likely to act appropriately, and thus success in action increases with the expenditure of less effort. The mind becomes quieter and is able to focus on its tasks. This smooth flow of energy makes meditative practices more fulfilling. In these circumstances, the healing potential within the body is at its greatest, stress can be released, and tissue repair quickened dramatically.

LEFT *The crown chakra.*

CROWN CHAKRA LAYOUT

During crystal healing sessions, it is common practice to place a clear quartz crystal close to the top of the head in the same way that a grounding stone is automatically placed near the feet. Clear quartz will add an extra dimension of order and brightness to the energy passing through the crown. With both these channels open and balanced, the body is free to absorb those qualities of energy most suited to its healing at that time.

Because of its holistic character, stones of other sorts may be discovered to balance the crown chakra, although the following suggestion will provide a good basis for most individual needs. Use three clear quartz crystals and place one centrally at the top of the head and one on each side. If the stones have points, direct them outward. You can add stones to this layout if you feel it is necessary.

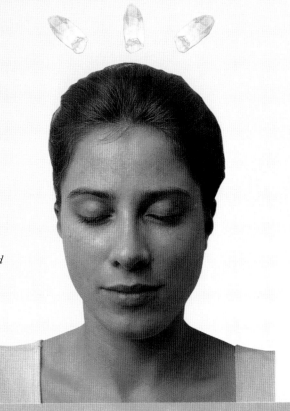

RIGHT *Clear quartz placed around the head helps to balance the crown chakra.*

Minor Chakras

In addition to the seven main chakras, there are numerous other energy centers that are located within and around the body, each with very specific functions.

There is a series of chakra points continuing along the body midline both above and below the physical points. The five chakras located above the head, numbered from 8 to 12, are related to universal and multidimensional vibrations. They are quite easy to locate by using a sensitized hand or a pendulum. When it is necessary to work with crystals on some of these upper five chakras, it normally signifies that some help is needed with information input into the conscious levels of the self.

The chakras located below the base of the spine—both midline and on the body at the knees, ankles, and feet—all work with aspects of physical existence, such as practical support, flexibility, and the relationship of self to surroundings. All of these chakra points can be used as alternative grounding positions. The chakra located just below the feet—the earth star chakra—is an especially powerful anchor point into this reality.

There are as many chakras to be found outside the physical body, within the aura, as there are on the body. Stones that are placed a considerable distance from the body can still have a profound effect and are often felt to be very powerful by the person being treated.

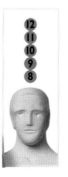

LEFT *The five upper chakras are associated with the vibrations held in the aura surrounding us.*

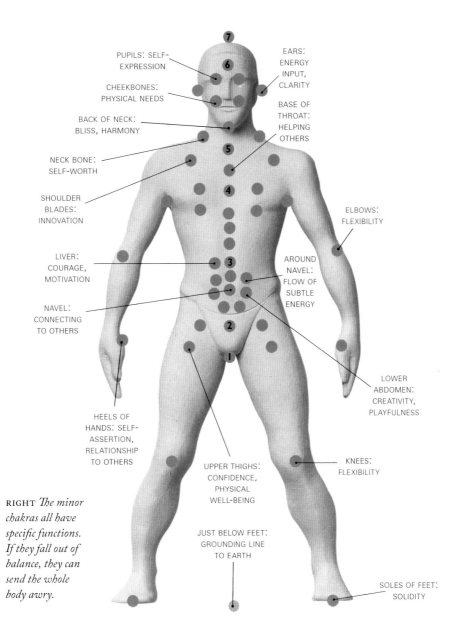

PUPILS: SELF-
EXPRESSION

EARS:
ENERGY
INPUT,
CLARITY

CHEEKBONES:
PHYSICAL NEEDS

BASE OF
THROAT:
HELPING
OTHERS

BACK OF NECK:
BLISS, HARMONY

NECK BONE:
SELF-WORTH

SHOULDER
BLADES:
INNOVATION

ELBOWS:
FLEXIBILITY

LIVER:
COURAGE,
MOTIVATION

AROUND
NAVEL:
FLOW OF
SUBTLE
ENERGY

NAVEL:
CONNECTING
TO OTHERS

LOWER
ABDOMEN:
CREATIVITY,
PLAYFULNESS

HEELS OF
HANDS: SELF-
ASSERTION,
RELATIONSHIP
TO OTHERS

UPPER THIGHS:
CONFIDENCE,
PHYSICAL
WELL-BEING

KNEES:
FLEXIBILITY

RIGHT *The minor
chakras all have
specific functions.
If they fall out of
balance, they can
send the whole
body awry.*

JUST BELOW FEET:
GROUNDING LINE
TO EARTH

SOLES OF FEET:
SOLIDITY

Simple Chakra Balances

Become familiar with the chakra positions and their primary associated colors and functions by starting off with simple healing exercises using a few crystals. Remember that the aim is to restore a normal functioning balance to the whole system.

Haphazard activation or focus on any one chakra can lead to serious imbalance on many levels—physical, emotional, mental, and spiritual. Learning and practicing spiritual exercises regularly, using crystals and other methods to alleviate stress and promote health, will naturally and safely enhance the quality of experience and the energy available within the body's systems.

Chakra Balance 1

Use clear quartz crystals, either natural or tumbled stones, of roughly the same size and weight. Place one on each chakra point and leave them for three or four minutes. After this time, remove all stones and simply lie relaxed for a few moments more. You may feel there is a need for a grounding stone to be placed between the feet. When you are doing these exercises by yourself, it is helpful to lay the stones out next to where you will be lying down. It is then much easier to place each stone without the others falling off.

Sometimes a stone will continually slip out of place. If this happens more than a couple of times, leave it where it has come to rest. Often the body has recognized a more appropriate placement for the stone and has made small movements to relocate it.

Some stones will feel extremely heavy, almost sinking into the body, while others will feel so light that they won't be noticed. Some stones may feel very cold, others burning hot, or itchy or even electric. You may also feel as if you are floating above the ground, or there may be a sensation of energy moving through the body or visual impressions of colors or patterns. All of these are natural as the body systems find their new equilibrium or release long-held stress and tensions.

A crystal healing session may be the first opportunity a person has had to relax completely while they are still awake. Feedback allows the healer to give reassurance.

Chakra Balance 2

Place clear quartz crystals, points inward, next to each side of the body at the level of each chakra. Here all stones are off the body, confirming that the sensations and experiences have been caused by a change in the energy flow rather than by the weight or temperature of the stones.

A variation on this balance is to first place the crystals with their points facing outward, releasing stress and tension. After three or four minutes, reverse the direction, so the points are now facing inward to recharge and energize the centers. After a few minutes, move the stones away from the body and rest a while. Use a grounding stone if necessary.

These are some techniques to practice on another person. They will encourage reliance on intuitive decisions as well as familiarity with the sequence of color and chakra *(see also page 120).*

Technique I: Choosing the Most Appropriate Stones

Placing a stone of the related color onto a chakra point, i.e. a light blue stone onto the throat center, has the effect of reinforcing the general qualities present there. This helps stimulate and balance the overall functions of each chakra but does not necessarily directly remove imbalances. In order to focus healing energy specifically on the areas needing attention, it may be that a crystal of another color is the best choice. A good assessment technique or well-tuned intuition is needed to work in this way.

RAINBOW SEQUENCE

At the crown chakra (7), place a white or clear stone, such as clear quartz. Golden or violet stones could also be used, such as amethyst, gold, or lemon quartz.

The third chakra, the solar plexus (3), has a yellow stone, such as citrine quartz, tiger's eye, pyrites, amber, or topaz.

In the center of the forehead at the brow chakra (6), use a dark blue or violet stone, such as lapis lazuli, sodalite, fluorite, or amethyst.

The sacral chakra (2) is balanced by an orange stone, such as carnelian, orange calcite, or a dark citrine quartz.

At the throat chakra (5) just above the sternal notch, place a light blue stone, such as blue lace agate, turquoise, or aquamarine.

Begin with a red stone, such as garnet or jasper, for the base chakra (1), placed either between the legs or two similar stones on the groin points.

At the heart chakra (4), place a green stone, such as jade, aventurine, bloodstone, or malachite. A small pink stone could be added.

Place a dark citrine, smoky quartz, hematite, or black tourmaline by the feet to stabilize and ground all the energies.

Using intuition alone, move to each chakra center and, with the palm of the hand or a crystal held in the hand, open your awareness to the energies present and intend that you will recognize any imbalances that are ready, willing, and able to be released safely and effectively. It is not necessary to be aware of this information at a conscious level. When you feel ready, move over to your healing crystals and pick up the first one that attracts your attention. Whatever the mineral or color, this will be the stone that will balance that chakra.

Repeat the intuitive process for each of the six remaining main chakras and then wait attentively for a few minutes more, watching for any signals to change, or remove the stones.

When the stones are all removed, settle the aura—sweep your hands slowly from head to feet with the clear intention to settle all energies to a normal functioning level, protecting and securing chakras and subtle bodies.

Technique II: Assessed Balance

Dowsing or muscle testing can be used in a similar way. Begin as always by centering and grounding your energies.

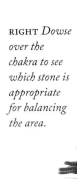

RIGHT *Dowse over the chakra to see which stone is appropriate for balancing the area.*

Dowse over each chakra center to determine which stone will best balance each area. Use color categories to narrow down the identification in the first instance. First, ask if it is a warm-colored stone (red, pink, orange, yellow) or a cool-colored (green, turquoise, blue, indigo, violet). If your testing indicates neither of these categories, ask about white, clear, black, or multicolored. The second question will identify the exact color of the stone needed—for example, pink.

The third question will identify which one of the pink minerals you have is the most appropriate to use. If you have more than one example of the crystal, a fourth question may identify one particular stone as being more effective than another of the same variety. This is not always necessary, but some bodies can be very fussy!

This way of working is much faster than to describe once the above pattern of questions is clear in your mind.

When all stones are in place, dowse for the length of time they need to remain on the body. Remove the stones and settle the aura as before.

Technique III: Single Spectrum

As a variation to this balance, begin by placing a single color stone on each chakra: red at base, orange at sacral, yellow at solar plexus, and so on. This will settle down the energy system and begin the healing process of the body. Once this is done, go back to the base chakra and check whether another stone will be of use to further increase the effectiveness of the balance. Proceed as with Techniques I or II. Particularly when you are learning crystal healing, it can take a while to work out which stones go where. For example, beginning with a basic chakra spectrum layout, or another simple calming and balancing layout *(see pages 72–73)*, while you are finding out what is required, increases the efficiency of the session and allows more profound healing to take place.

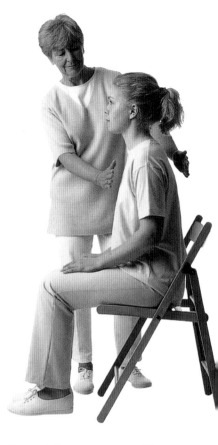

ABOVE *Select a stone of related color and place it on the chakra point you are going to work on.*

Technique IV: Balancing Chakras for Over- and Under- Energy

We have seen how an intuitive approach can identify and balance any chakras that are overenergized or lacking in energy. Exactly the same procedure can be adapted to the use of assessment by pendulum or muscle- testing.

Check if it is appropriate to balance the body for over- and under- energies with the following steps:

1. Move to each chakra in turn. Ask the question: "Is this chakra balanced?"

2. If the answer is "yes," ask whether it requires a stone to maintain its balance while you are working on the remaining chakras.

3. If the chakra is out of balance, the next questions will be: "Is this chakra underenergized? Is this chakra overenergized?"

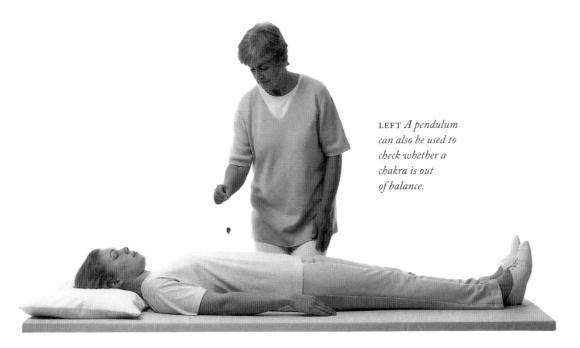

LEFT *A pendulum can also be used to check whether a chakra is out of balance.*

STRUCTURE AND INTUITION

In a learning situation, it is vital to begin with a clearly discernible working structure within which personal experiences can be firmly set or measured. Time and again I have watched trainee healers flounder simply because they place no confidence in their own intuitive abilities. Intuition flourishes when there is stability and confidence. It withers away when there is doubt about ability. Structure provides the relaxation within which personal skills can begin to mature.

4. Next, identify, using color and type categories, which crystal will restore the chakra to normal, balanced function.

5. Check whether additional crystals are needed, in the case of under energy, to direct energy toward the chakra or, for over energy, to lead it away from the area. Use quartz points or other crystals with strong direction to help restore a balance of energy. Tourmaline, topaz, kyanite, kunzite, selenite, and all stones with parallel striations tend to be good energy shifters.

6. Remove the stones. Dowse first in order to find out whether the order of the stones' removal is important. Sometimes extra or directional stones are best removed first, before the main chakra stones are taken away. This makes the whole process a smoother experience.

RIGHT *The parallel striations on tourmaline make it a good energy shifter.*

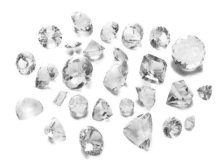

Color Meditation for Assessing Chakras

*T*he imaginative skills of the mind can provide the crystal healer with many ways to recognize and assess energy patterns within the subtle anatomy. Unexpected images and feelings are an indication that your mind has gone beyond the stage of guided visualization and is really perceiving with some accuracy what is actually present on subtle levels. Often the awareness initially needs to be pointed in the right direction. Guided visualization, imagining, or "pretending" sets the scene and helps establish a state of passive attentiveness in which the everyday conscious mind drops some of its analytical hold on what is perceived.

The Uses of Guided Visualization

Often your awareness initially needs to be pointed in the right direction. The more familiar your mind becomes with a repeated sequence of images, or instruction, the easier it is to slip into a receptive frame of mind where intuition can arise, and the visualization takes on a life of its own.

Body Viewing/Body Overview

This exercise in visualization allows someone to scan their body in a way that may suggest which areas are in need of balancing and healing.

1. After grounding and centering your energies, and totally relaxing your physical body, imagine that you are looking at an image of yourself. It might be a mirror image or a picture, or you might see if you can move away from where you are lying and then turn around to look at yourself. Or you may visualize yourself floating upward and then looking down on your resting body.

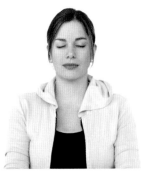

ABOVE *The key to using guided visualization and body overview methods is to be attentive and receptive to what comes into your mind.*

The image does not need to be photographically clear; a faint impression will do to start.

2. Now take a look over, in, and around your body image. There may be areas of color, or light and shade, or you may find it difficult to see some parts.

3. Wherever there is a darker area, or turbulence of some kind, or a lack of definition, gently focus on that with your subtle senses. Be aware of any emotional content or any thoughts that arise. These may indicate the causes of disturbance and the crystals that will help rebalance the body.

4. It is not necessary to become intensely attached to what you see. This is simply a quick glance using fine levels of the sense perceptions to identify and

DRAWING DOWN COLORS

This meditation can be fully visualized and elaborate, or carried out very quickly, drawing colors one after the other to the chakras and down to the ground. The exercise strengthens each chakra center with its balancing color vibration. You may notice that some parts seem easier to imagine than others. Some chakras might seem never to get filled. This will give some indication as to which energy centers may need more attention. Any area difficult to visualize needs more work to integrate it fully into the whole system. This technique can be a useful diagnostic tool.

1 *Make sure you are seated comfortably. Center and ground yourself and then imagine a large bright sphere of white light suspended above your head.*

2 *From this sphere, you will be able to draw down any color at will.*

3 *Imagine a good, strong red light in the sphere. Pull it down into your body and down the spine to fill up the base chakra with deep, red energy. Allow the color to fill the chakra and let any overflow pass down into the Earth.*

4 *Take orange from the sphere. Let it sink down to the sacral chakra, the hara, the center of gravity between the pelvic bones. Let the orange fill the area and allow any excess to drain away into the Earth.*

deal with areas of imbalance. Unless you have already set mental parameters, your vision will include all energy levels, from the physical to the highest spiritual body, so avoid analysis and the temptation to diagnose.

The technique below will give you an indication of the state of your chakras, while at the same time strengthening the energy of each with the appropriate color. Any area that seems more difficult to imagine with clarity may indicate some lack of energy there, so spend a little more time focusing color into that spot.

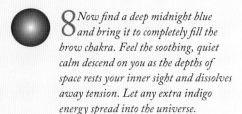 *5 Now return to the white light sphere and let yellow stream down to your solar plexus. Let it gather there until it becomes like a bright sun that illuminates the whole of your body. Take time to make sure there are no areas left in shadow. Allow any excess to flow into the Earth.*

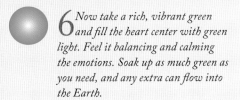 *6 Now take a rich, vibrant green and fill the heart center with green light. Feel it balancing and calming the emotions. Soak up as much green as you need, and any extra can flow into the Earth.*

7 Take a sky-blue light from the sphere above you and flood the throat center with cool - blue radiance. See the blue flow in and all around you, forging links of information and understanding with the world. Let the extra energy sweep right through you into the Earth.

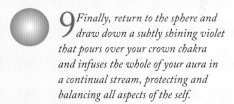 *8 Now find a deep midnight blue and bring it to completely fill the brow chakra. Feel the soothing, quiet calm descend on you as the depths of space rests your inner sight and dissolves away tension. Let any extra indigo energy spread into the universe.*

9 Finally, return to the sphere and draw down a subtly shining violet that pours over your crown chakra and infuses the whole of your aura in a continual stream, protecting and balancing all aspects of the self.

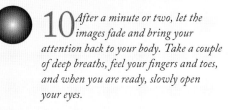 *10 After a minute or two, let the images fade and bring your attention back to your body. Take a couple of deep breaths, feel your fingers and toes, and when you are ready, slowly open your eyes.*

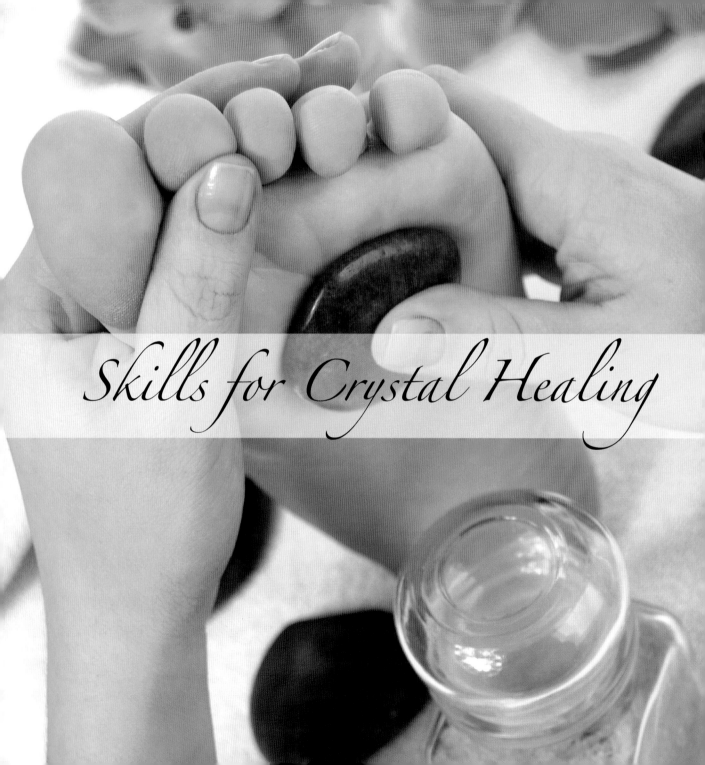

Skills for Crystal Healing

Pendulum Dowsing

A pendulum is any balanced weight suspended by a chain or thread and is simply a means of visibly checking what the unconscious mind already knows. The pendulum represents an extension of the inner senses and creates a visual representation of inner energy changes. The pendulum amplifies small muscle movements that result from changes in subtle energy flow through the physical body. The conscious mind, emotions, and physical tension can all affect the pendulum.

ABOVE *Pendulums used for dowsing will need occasional cleaning.*

When there is an emotional investment in the answer, dowsing will nearly always produce an unreliable result. The skill in effective pendulum dowsing is to remain in a relaxed, neutral frame of mind and to have a good system of questioning. When dowsing, it is a good idea to check your positive and negative responses each time the pendulum is used. It is also a good idea to check any new pendulum you might use.

BELOW *The body's energy flow is reflected in pendulum movement. You need to be relaxed before starting.*

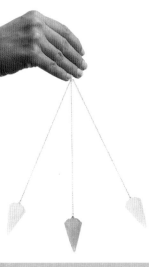

Techniques for Pendulum Dowsing

Pendulum assessment is only as accurate as the questioning techniques used. Effective dowsing requires entering an altered state of awareness slightly removed from everyday processes. It is a delicate state to maintain, and the following guidelines may be helpful:

1. Center and ground your energies before you begin assessments.

2. Check the "yes" or "no" swings of your pendulum.

3. Confirm that you are ready, willing, and able to carry out the assessment work. If there is a negative response here, check whether you need to do something else first.

AN INTRODUCTION TO PENDULUM DOWSING

PENDULUM PROCEDURE

1 *Choose a pendulum with which you feel comfortable. It should be well-balanced and feel neither too heavy nor too light. Use either hand.*

2 *Keep the string, chain, or thread about 4 or 5 inches (10–12 cm) long. Hold the pendulum between your thumb and index finger. Hold your forearm parallel to the ground, with your wrist relaxed.*

3 *Set the pendulum in a gentle, neutral swing, moving in a straight line away from you. Let it swing about eight times to get the feel of it. Bring it to a halt either by stopping it with your other hand or by using a small upward jerk of the hand.*

4 *Repeat the neutral swing to begin, and after a short time mentally ask the pendulum to begin to develop into a clockwise, circular, or elliptical motion for another six to eight rotations. Stop the pendulum again.*

5 *Repeat the exercise; this time ask the pendulum to make a counterclockwise movement.*

6 *When you are confident with these exercises, use your intention to stop the pendulum and keep it still.*

PENDULUM RESPONSES

Before you start, use a grounding and centering technique *(see pages 53–64).* It is good practice to get into the habit of automatically balancing your energies before beginning. Next, find out in which direction the pendulum will move in response to "yes" and "no" answers. "Yes" and "no" responses are entirely individual. Some people have circular swings, and some elliptical, some directional straight lines.

RESPONSE PROCEEDURE

1 *Hold your free hand over your solar plexus and set the pendulum into a neutral swing to tap into your own energy systems directly.*

2 *Without focusing on the movement of the pendulum, ask for it to move in a direction that indicates a "yes" response.*

3 *Once a strong swing becomes clear, make a note of the type of swing and its direction.*

4 *Stop the pendulum.*

5 *Repeat, asking to be shown a "no" response.*

6 *Repeat this process until you are confident in the responses.*

Always ask questions or make statements in the simplest language and make sure that they can be answered with a "yes" or "no." Where there is a question with significant emotional loading for the questioner—that is, there is an obvious preferred outcome—neutrality can be slightly enhanced by clearly stating "yes" or "no" after the question.

Dowsing with Lists and Arcs

Mental and emotional neutrality can be easier to maintain if dowsing is done with lists, arcs, or with your free hand touching or pointing to stones. Lists can be made of anything useful to the healer. They can be specific, such as chakras, meridians, or types of stone, or general, such as colors or numbers. A number list, for example, can be used to find out how long a stone needs to be in place, how often a stone needs cleansing, and so on.

All questioning should start off with big categories and work down to small areas. For example, "Does this chakra require a warm-colored stone?" The response immediately narrows the search to either red-orange-yellow or green-blue-violet areas. It works similarly with timing or amounts. Use the phrase "more than..." i.e. "Does this stone need to be in position for more than ten minutes?"

Use lists in the same way, beginning with large categories, such as: "Is this list appropriate?", "Is this what is needed?" With your free hand, touch or define what you are asking about.

Dowsing arcs are used instead of circles because any pendulum swing on a circle will pick out two sections at the top and bottom of the swing, but only one possible section is indicated on an arc.

DOWSING WITH ARCS

- Ground and center yourself *(see pages 53–64)*.

- Place the dowsing arc in front of you on a flat surface.

- Touch the arc and ask if this arc is appropriate. If it is, ask the pendulum to swing in a line to indicate the appropriate answer. Keep the pendulum fairly close to the flat surface so that it is easier to identify the correct section.

- Let the pendulum move in a straight swing from the central point where you are keeping it. When the pendulum settles to a new angle of swing, check the response by placing a finger of your free hand on the segment and use the yes or no procedure. It is wise to avoid focusing on the pendulum until its angle has stabilized. The eye can hold back the movement by its concentration at an inappropriate location.

- Always get into the habit of asking: "Is there anything else?" You should not assume you have all the answers when more information might be available.

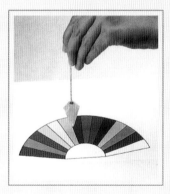

ABOVE *Dowsing arcs can be divided into several sections. For example, an arc divided into color sections can help the healer decide which colored stone is most appropriate to use.*

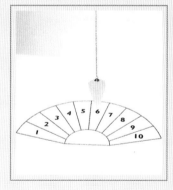

ABOVE *Dowsing arcs divided into numbers will help answer any questions regarding timing and quantity. A list of numbers can be just as effective.*

Assessment Using Kinesiology

Kinesiology, commonly known as muscle testing, is perhaps one of the most useful assessment tools any healer can learn. Essentially, muscle testing is an extension of the same processes that allow pendulum dowsing to work—that is, the physical body responds clearly to very small changes of energy flow within its subtle systems. Every stimulus, whether it comes from the sense organs, a verbal cue, or a thought or emotion, affects the quality of life energy, either enhancing or depleting it.

Kinesiology testing arose when chiropractors noticed that a muscle would tend to have less tone when held in certain positions or when other points on the body were touched. This observation was developed into a coherent assessment and healing system by applying muscle groups to the main energy meridians identified in traditional Chinese medicine. Responses in certain muscles would indicate that a particular meridian was either strong or weak.

In crystal healing, the most useful muscle-testing techniques deal mainly with a "yes" or "no" response. The advantage of using muscle testing is that it involves the patient. It is their own body that responds to questions about what methods of healing would be the most useful. It is very apparent when a muscle tests strong and when it tests weak. It can be a clear demonstration, for example, that a certain crystal dramatically increases the available life energy. A healer using a pendulum may obtain the same degree of accuracy as from muscle testing, but having a choice of tools increases a healer's flexibility.

The accuracy of muscle testing depends upon a baseline of grounded and centered energy where there is stability and focus and a carefully maintained mental neutrality. Any stress factors are likely to disrupt temporarily the baseline energy of either the healer or the patient. This is known as switching—where responses to some questions become random and inaccurate.

Always begin all testing by tapping in or using other grounding and centering exercises *(see pages 53–64)*. Repeat these procedures where switching is suspected. Use muscle testing to check every stage of corrective work for its effectiveness.

Healing is always a joining and understanding between healer and patient. Belief systems and preconceived ideas become part of a circuit of merged energies, which cannot be avoided. However, a confident attitude, humor, self-awareness, and humility all reduce the chance of deception.

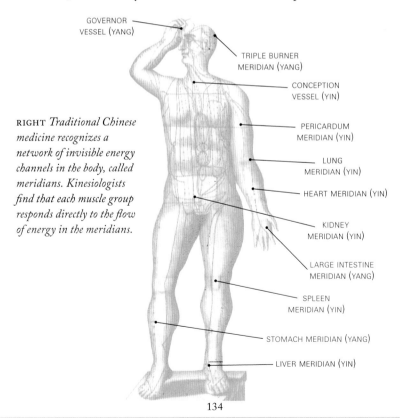

GOVERNOR VESSEL (YANG)

TRIPLE BURNER MERIDIAN (YANG)

CONCEPTION VESSEL (YIN)

PERICARDUM MERIDIAN (YIN)

LUNG MERIDIAN (YIN)

HEART MERIDIAN (YIN)

KIDNEY MERIDIAN (YIN)

LARGE INTESTINE MERIDIAN (YANG)

SPLEEN MERIDIAN (YIN)

STOMACH MERIDIAN (YANG)

LIVER MERIDIAN (YIN)

RIGHT *Traditional Chinese medicine recognizes a network of invisible energy channels in the body, called meridians. Kinesiologists find that each muscle group responds directly to the flow of energy in the meridians.*

General Muscle Testing

The key with muscle testing is to feel the response in the muscles on which you are working. Every person is different, so you will need to practice to find the appropriate level of testing for an individual. Both people should be relaxed before you begin. Use minimal physical effort *(see step 1 on page 136)*.

Here we are simply concerned with using muscle testing as an indicator. Any muscle test can be used as an indicator, but some are easier to use and less tiring.

Testing can be carried out standing, sitting, or lying down, but make sure the body is not lopsided, the hands are not touching the body, and the legs are uncrossed. Make sure other muscle groups are not being used to strengthen the test. If you make sure that both of you are not holding your breath when testing, or are both gently breathing out, this will help prevent tensing.

Muscles to Test:

Anterior deltoid

Start by holding the arm straight out at an angle of 35 degrees. The elbow should be locked, palm down. The movement is straight downward. The tester should use light downward pressure, located just above the wrist.

Brachioradialis

The upper arm is held close to the body, lower arm bent at an angle of about 35 degrees with palm toward the body. The movement is straight down. This is usually an easy test, since it doesn't need much effort and isn't too tiring.

Anterior serratus

A stronger muscle test than the previous one but can be less tiring when lying down. The arm is held upright at 90 degrees to the body, palm facing down toward the feet. The movement is straight down along the line of the body.

Latissiumus dorsi

This muscle must be tested very lightly with two fingers only. The arm is held straight, elbow locked tight to the side with palm facing outward. The tester pulls gently away from the body just above the wrist *(see box below)*.

MUSCLE TESTING

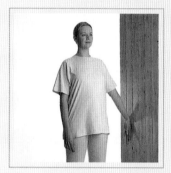

1 *Stand a little way from a wall so that if you raise your arm, you will touch it. Feel your muscles activating as you push forward gently against the surface. This is all the pressure you should be using in testing others.*

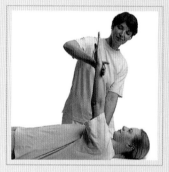

2 *Demonstrate the movement of the limb with your partner. Move your partner's arm through the range of movements to show the direction and muscles being used. This picture shows the anterior serratus muscle being tested.*

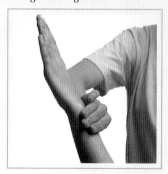

3 *Put the limb into position and say "hold." When carrying out a test, stay away from pulse points and do not grip the arm. Use a flat palm or two or three fingers held straight.*

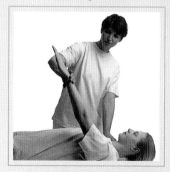

4 *Pause for a second and then evenly and gradually apply enough pressure to see whether the muscle locks or feels weak and spongy. After a couple of seconds, gently and gradually release the pressure.*

Other Hints for Muscle Testing

• Always support the arm once it has been tested. Leaving it in the air or letting it drop is very tiring.

• If tests are weak, have the person drink some water, and then retest.

• If a result is unclear, repeat the test. A weak muscle will become progressively weaker; a strong muscle will strengthen further.

• Ask the person how a test feels if you are not sure whether a muscle is strong or weak.

• There are degrees of weakness: no resistance at all, slow weakening, hesitant weakness, or a spongy feeling. Many people's arms will move some distance before locking. This distance needs gauging in each person. If you continue to be unsure of the responses, either use self-testing surrogate techniques or change to pendulum dowsing.

• Keep your tone of voice constant when making statements. Do not favor one possibility over any other.

• Don't stare or maintain long eye contact, because this reduces the emotional and mental neutrality essential for good results.

• If muscles on one side of the body are weak or tired, try those on the other side. Muscles eventually tire too much to continue testing.

• If responses become confused or don't make sense, it is usually a sign of switching *(see box on page 138)*. Tap in to restore balance. Important, traumatic, or emotional issues are likely to cause switching.

RIGHT *Test for the anterior deltoid muscle. Remember to support the patient's arm as you work and avoid pulse points. Keep your hand flat.*

TEST FOR SWITCHING

Now that you have a strong indicator muscle, it is necessary to check whether
the body is in sufficient balance to test accurately that it is not switched.
The following are four quick pre-tests to carry out:

1 *Ask your partner to place the palm of their free hand over their navel. Test the muscle again. If the muscle test remains strong, continue to step 2.*

2 *Put the tip of one finger on any muscle and test. This time, the muscle test should be weak. Repeat the test with the tips of two adjacent fingers on any muscle. Now the muscle should test strong.*

3 *Now lightly pinch the center of any muscle. This should weaken your test muscle. Smooth over the muscle, and the test should now be strong.*

4 *Silently or out loud say "yes" and test the muscle. It should stay strong. Then say "no" and test the muscle. It should be weak. Now the muscle test has clearly indicated that the body can react to both positive and negative states. Continue with your assessment. If any test did not produce the correct response, tap in the body and repeat the tests. These switching tests are checking that the body is, first, in general balance with all its meridians, or energy pathways, and second, that it recognizes electromagnetic polarity. Different areas of the body carry different electrical charges—some areas positively and some negatively charged. The test means the body is recognizing these polarities accurately. Third, it checks that the nerve impulses to and from the brain are working correctly and, last, that the body recognizes the difference between positive and negative statements.*

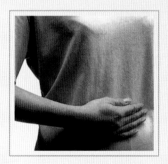

ABOVE *Test for switching by asking your partner to put their palm over their navel while you test the indicator muscle.*

SELF-TESTING AND SURROGATE TESTING

Self-testing is a useful technique to muscle test yourself as an alternative to pendulum dowsing. It can also be used in surrogate testing. This is where the tester keeps in physical contact with the patient to ensure a flow of information and energy and asks questions of the patient via the tester's own energy system.

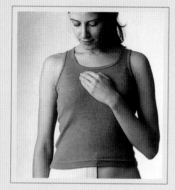

1 As with all forms of muscle testing, begin the session by grounding, centering, and tapping in (see pages 53–64).

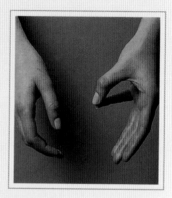

2 Let the tips of both thumb and little finger of the left hand touch.

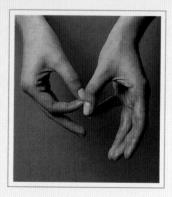

3 Now insert the thumb and index finger of the right hand with tips touching into the gap between the palm of the left hand and the thumb and little finger of the left hand.

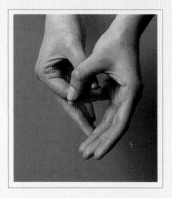

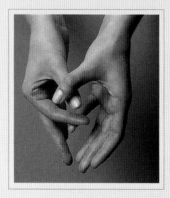

4 By parting the thumb and index finger of the right hand sharply outward to contact the thumb and finger of the left hand, you are testing the muscles that are responsible for keeping the left-hand fingertip and thumb together.

5 If the fingertips of the left hand stay in contact, or move only slightly apart and then lock, the energy is still flowing through the muscles, and for most people this indicates a "yes" response.

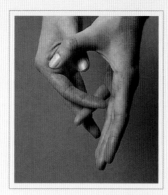

6 If the fingertips of the left hand part appreciably, the muscles have weakened, and for most people this is a "no" response.

Learning to Sense the Auric Field

*W*orking with crystals naturally seems to increase the sensitivity to subtle energy fields, and there are many ways to explore and increase this ability. Everyone is familiar with receiving information from nonconscious levels of awareness. It is a normal part of functioning as a human being and such a natural skill that it is rarely given much thought.

We all have a sense of personal space, an area around us that we feel belongs to us. Intrusions into this space make us feel uncomfortable and threatened, although closeness with those we like does not present any problems at all. What is being experienced here may be some sort of disharmony between auric fields. Similarly, many of us will notice a change of atmosphere when certain people enter a room, even when we are not aware of the fact because we are looking in another direction.

Recent experimentation also clearly suggests that, at some unconscious level, we are aware of being stared at by someone hidden from view. It is frequently the case that students of subtle energies become discouraged because they cannot see auras. Subtle sight is one of the last skills to develop, and one that requires great skill to interpret correctly. At the level of feeling, with a mixture of intuition, emotion, and empathy, nearly everyone can achieve usable results with a little practice.

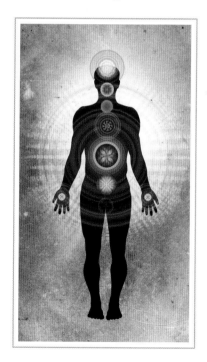

SENSITIVITY EXERCISE 1

First it is necessary to turn our attention toward the energy feeling of our own bodies. One of the easiest methods is to rub the palms of the hands together vigorously. Separate your hands and then from a distance bring them toward each other.

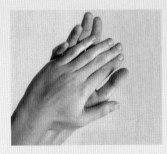

RUB PALMS
TOGETHER
VIGOROUSLY

At a certain point, there will be a sensation of pressure, a thickening of the air. There will be a feeling of pressure somewhere within the physical body, not necessarily in the hands, that could be described as heat, tickling, or itching, like static electricity. These differences of body sensation and emotional feeling are our responses to energy fields. Continue gently contracting and expanding the space between your hands. You may find that the force builds up and increases in size and that it becomes quite difficult to push your palms together. When you have experimented enough, relax and breathe the energy back into your body. The Chinese describe this chi energy as having the consistency of thick honey, so your receptivity will increase with slow, even movements.

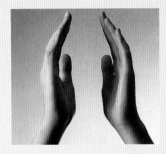

PUSH HANDS
TOGETHER FROM
A DISTANCE

SENSITIVITY EXERCISE 2

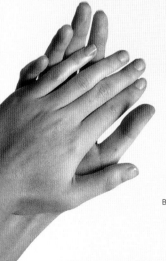

Try the same experiment with the hands after rubbing a crystal between your palms. What difference does this make to your sensitivity? Use a small clear quartz crystal and then try out different sorts of stone, such as tumbled varieties of quartz: rose, rutilated, citrine, tiger's eye, or aventurine. Make a note of any differences you notice between the different stones.

RUB A CRYSTAL
BETWEEN THE PALMS

SENSITIVITY EXERCISE 3

Now, with sensitized hands, slowly approach other objects. See where you notice a change of feeling within your body. Try it with a plant, a book, a crystal, and another person. You should notice that the fields extend different distances away from animate and inanimate objects or person.

Always remember to center and ground yourself before starting so that you are clear about which sensations are yours and which you are picking up from the object or person.

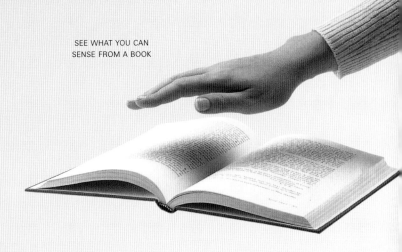

SEE WHAT YOU CAN SENSE FROM A BOOK

EVERYTHING POSSESSES AN ENERGY FIELD, WHETHER IT IS ANIMATE OR INANIMATE

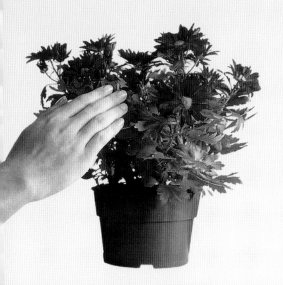

Take time to experiment with hand dowsing. With practice, it is possible to receive other types of information when you link into these energy fields. Listening to your body in this way will greatly enhance your intuitive abilities at the same time as focusing away from the conscious, chattering, everyday mind.

Pay attention to any physical sensations as well as any changes in your emotions or thought patterns. If you are unsure of what you are feeling, move away and slowly back again. You should notice the same sorts of changes as the aura is encountered.

Working with Intuition

*W*orking with intuition requires a light touch and a sense of play. Begin these procedures by grounding and centering your energies. Working at this level of intuition can create a slightly more dissociative state than other methods, so grounding must he maintained throughout.

Balancing the Chakras

This method requires a slightly more detailed intuitive assessment of the state of each chakra. Here we want to establish if a chakra is underenergized or overenergized. This means identifying if the energy balance within each chakra is adequate to deal with its current energy requirements. Both over energized and underenergized states may create compensatory imbalances in other chakra centers in order to restore equilibrium.

Under energy is often felt as coolness, hollowness, a dip in energy, a lack of some kind. Over energy usually seems to be a pressure, turbulence, heat, buildup, or excess of some sort. Where you come across stress or a need for healing energy, you may have a sense of discomfort or a feeling that something is out of place. This may be happening on many different levels—don't assume that it can be identified as a physical problem. Even if it is a very strong subjective experience, this doesn't necessarily mean the imbalance is large or significant. It may merely show that it is close to the surface or that you will be able to release it easily.

You may wish to check whether any physical symptoms have occurred in the areas that feel disturbed, but do not cause worry. Crystal healing recognizes the imbalances that can be dealt with safely at any one time. As crystal healing concerns the whole person, it isn't always possible to identify what is going on. The healer is simply helping the body to function more effectively and therefore more healthily.

INTUITIVE SELECTION

Be aware of what your body selects as the most appropriate crystals. It is helpful to know the areas of each crystal's use, but this is only a guideline. A stone will cause varying energy conditions as its vibratory pattern interfaces with those of different people.

INTUITIVE CHAKRA BALANCE

1 *After grounding and centering (see pages 53–64), frame the intent to balance the seven main chakras. Rub your hands together, or hold a crystal to stimulate sensitivity in your palms.*

2 *Make a quick upward sweep of the body, moving from the feet to the head.*

3 *Return to the base chakra. Hold your open palm over the area for a little while.*

4 *Move to where your stones are laid out and pick up the first one or two that draw your attention. Place them close to the base chakra.*

5 *Each time stones are placed, check the experiences of your patient.*

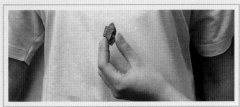

6 *Repeat this process for each of the main chakras. Do not be concerned about the color or type of stone. Your intention is to bring balance so that is what your intuition is helping to achieve.*

7 *When all chakras have one or more stones placed near them, stand back a little and look to see how it feels. Where the eyes settle repeatedly can often suggest that changes of some kind need to be made.*

8 *Leave the stones in place for about ten minutes, or less time if you have a strong feeling that the balance is complete.*

9 *Remove all stones and then scan each chakra again, this time with the clear intention of protecting and restoring each to normal functioning.*

10 *Talk over any experiences with your patient, as feedback is always useful.*

These are important exercises to practice. They can loosen up any tendencies to repeatedly use the same types of stones or corrections. Individual energy levels are unique, ever-changing, and far too complex for the conscious awareness of a healer to understand. Creating an intuitive link allows the precise needs of the body to be matched with the energy of a crystal.

RANDOM INTUITIVE LAYOUT

SWEEP YOUR
HAND OVER THE
AURIC FIELD

SUGILITE

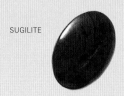

SELECT A STONE
AT RANDOM

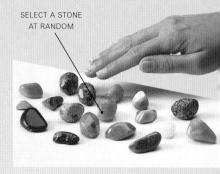

1 *Start by framing a clear intention to balance the energies of this person.*

2 *Take time to sweep your hand over the auric field of your patient. Begin at the feet and, holding your hand palm down, a few inches above the body, slowly move upward.*

3 *Be aware of any changes you may feel. This is allowing information concerning the energy status of the patient to register in your own subtle awareness. If you scan the entire body up to the head without feeling any particular sensations, it doesn't matter. Trust your body awareness.*

4 *Having completed the scan, move quickly to where all your stones have been laid out so that you can see them all at once. Don't worry if your collection isn't very big; your intuitive skills will select the most appropriate stone.*

AMBER

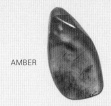

5 *Without thinking about their specific purpose, simply pick up those stones that attract your attention.*

6 *Return to the person's side and carefully place the stones anywhere on or around the body where it feels right.*

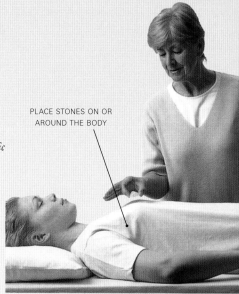

PLACE STONES ON OR
AROUND THE BODY

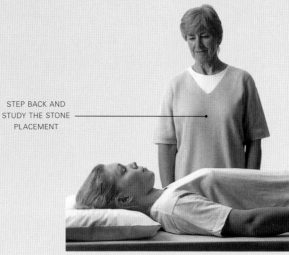

STEP BACK AND
STUDY THE STONE
PLACEMENT

7 Ignore any knowledge you might have about your patient's health or about their chakra and subtle bodies. The aim here is to work without engaging the analytical part of the brain.

8 Take no more than a minute to place all the stones.

9 Step back a little so that you can see the whole body easily. If you now feel unhappy about some crystal placements, move them to a different place or perhaps take them away completely.

10 Check how the patient feels to make sure there is no discomfort anywhere.

11 Continue to gaze gently over the crystal placements. If you feel that any changes are needed, make them.

12 Stay relaxed and attentive, and you will probably have a clear sense of when the stones need to he removed, but remove them all within ten minutes.

13 Repeat your hand scan and note any changes that have occurred.

14 Finish the scan with a couple of sweeps from head to feet, with the clear intention to normalize all functions and protect the auric integrity.

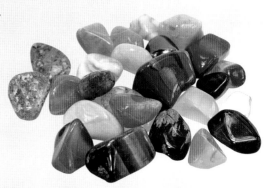

INTUITIVE PROCEDURE

Depending on your lifestyle and level of activity, some chakras will occasionally need to be more active than others. Here we are helping readjust inappropriate imbalances only.

1 Cleanse your stones, then ground and center yourself (see pages 29–32 and 53–64).

2 Frame the intent to help bring balance to any overactive or underactive chakras, then scan the midline of the body from feet to head. This can be done just with the hand, but your sensitivity may increase if you hold a comfortably large clear quartz crystal in your hand. Hold the crystal's point almost parallel to the body lying down and move it slowly up toward the head.

3 When you come to the area of a main chakra, pay attention to how it feels.

4 You may want to repeat this scanning several times to allow you to gauge the difference between various chakras.

5 Those chakras in balance will often not give much response. Your intent is to look for imbalances, so that is what your subtle senses will notice most. Those out of balance will feel distinctly different, depending upon the way your own body translates the energy patterns into sensation. Only practice and experience will teach you exactly how your senses react.

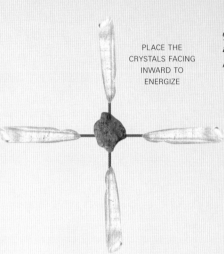

PLACE THE CRYSTALS FACING INWARD TO ENERGIZE

6 Having identified any chakras that are underenergized or overenergized, return to each one in turn. Hold your hand or crystal above the chakra to refamiliarize yourself with its energy state, then quickly select stones that draw your attention. Three or four may come up.

7 Lay the stones on the chakra in a way that feels right or comfortable.

8 Where there is under energy, use between two to four small, clear quartz crystals and place them around that area with points inward. This will help energize it.

9 Where there is over energy, once the intuited stones are in place, use small clear quartz stones with their points facing outward to release any excess buildup of energy.

10 If in adjacent chakras, one area is overenergized, and the other is underenergized, a clear quartz crystal can be placed with its point toward the under energy, thus helping balance out the centers.

11 It may feel appropriate to place one stone on each chakra, even those not out of balance. Within this procedural framework, follow your own intuitive feelings.

12 *After ten minutes, begin to remove the stones. Unless there is a clear sense to do otherwise, it is good policy to first remove all the energy-directing stones and then return to remove the chakra stones.*

13 *Repeat the scan with hand or crystal to check that all chakras feel equally energized.*

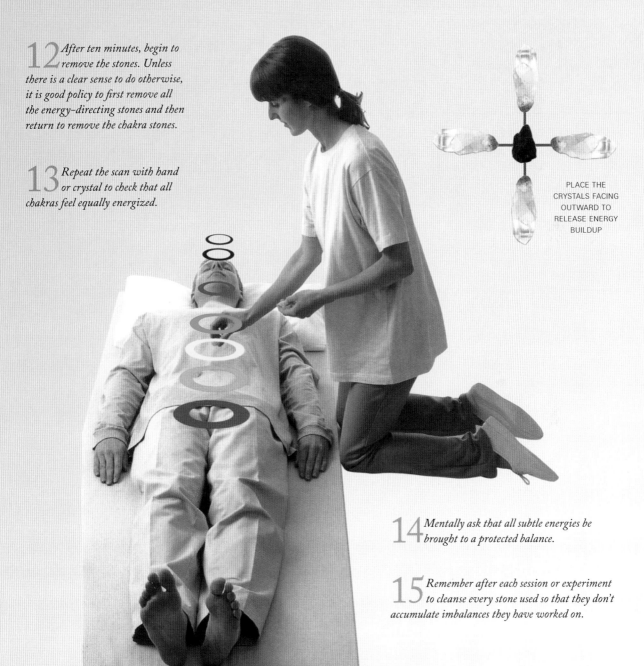

PLACE THE CRYSTALS FACING OUTWARD TO RELEASE ENERGY BUILDUP

14 *Mentally ask that all subtle energies be brought to a protected balance.*

15 *Remember after each session or experiment to cleanse every stone used so that they don't accumulate imbalances they have worked on.*

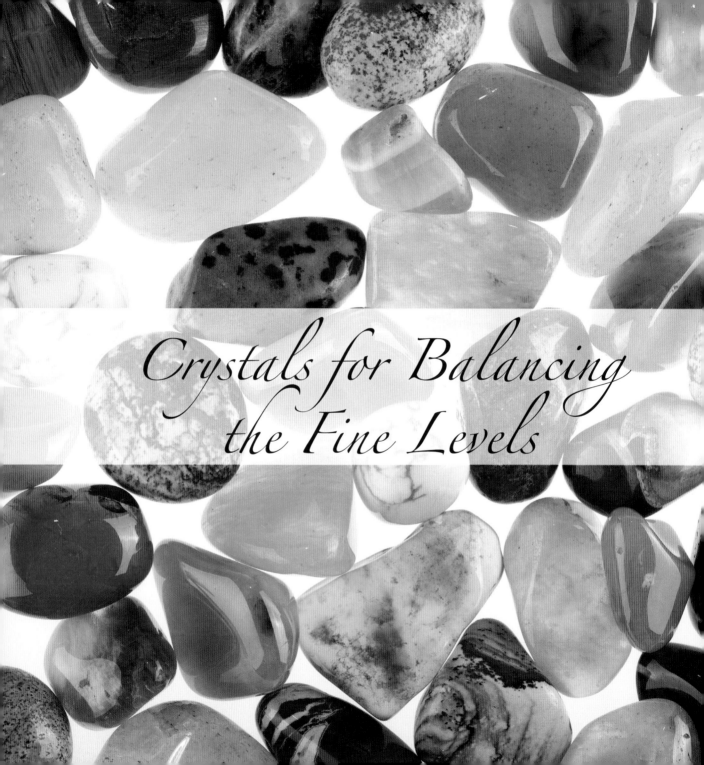

Crystals for Balancing the Fine Levels

Seven Subtle Bodies

Described here is a model of seven subtle bodies, each level extending further from the physical body and made of finer energy material. It is important to remember that each succeeding level interpenetrates all of the previous levels, including the physical, so that there is a continuous, dynamic, and complex interaction between them.

The Etheric Body

The etheric body is the closest to the physical, and it is considered to be the blueprint upon which the cells and organs are built. When imbalance and weakness occur in the etheric area, they will eventually manifest themselves on the physical level. The meridian system is believed to be integrated with the etheric body and to act as the interface between etheric and physical.

The Emotional Body

The emotional body is the container of feelings. It roughly follows the body's outline but extends further than the etheric. It is composed of colored clouds of energy that are in continual flux, altering according to mood and emotional state. This field is often the aura of colors that sensitives perceive around a person. The emotional body holds our psychological stability and our sensitivity to those around us.

The Mental Body

The mental body is associated with thoughts and mental processes. It is usually perceived as bright yellow, expanding around the head during mental concentration. In the mental body we interpret information according to the belief structures that we have developed since birth.

The Astral Body

The astral body is the fourth layer. This subtly colored energy layer contains the essence of our personality. It is the boundary layer between the current individual personality and a more collective spiritual awareness and is concerned with relationships, particularly these that encompass the whole of humanity.

The Causal, Soul, and Spiritual Bodies

The functions of the three remaining subtle bodies are not so clearly defined. The fifth layer is the causal body, which links the personality to the collective unconscious and is the doorway to higher levels of consciousness. The soul, or celestial, body is the sixth subtle level. It seems to focus fine levels of universal energy and is related to the idea of the Higher Self. The spiritual body is the seventh subtle body. It is the container and integrator of all other subtle energies. It has access to all universal energies but maintains the individuality of each being.

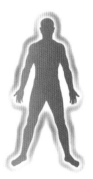 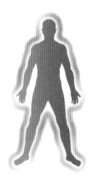 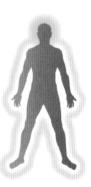 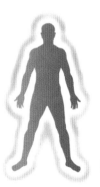 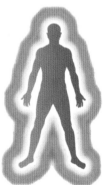

ETHERIC BODY   EMOTIONAL BODY   MENTAL BODY   ASTRAL BODY   SPIRITUAL BODIES

Crystal Layouts

*T*he following layouts work with particular subtle bodies. They may be used in healing situations or to familiarize yourself with each level of awareness. The better we understand our own energy, the less likely we are to misinterpret other people.

Physical Body Layout

Tourmaline is a crystal with many varied uses in healing. One of its most useful attributes is its ability to help repair the physical body, particularly structural problems in the bones or muscle tissue.

Black tourmaline grounds, protects, and integrates personal energy. Use eight black tourmaline crystals; tumbled stones or fragments will work almost as well. If the stones have natural terminations, they should be placed pointing toward the body. Create two intersecting rectangles. The first is made of four tourmalines: one above the head, one below the feet, one midway down the body next to each side. If you lie down with your head to north, the stones are aligned to the north, south, east, and west.

The second rectangle is made with the remaining four crystals placed about 20 to 25 degrees clockwise to the first stones, making a slightly offset rectangle. A green background will enhance the effects of this layout. Initially, there may be some increase in aches and pains, but these will diminish quite rapidly as the body gently realigns itself. If there are chronic skeletal problems, regular short exposure to this layout will prove most effective.

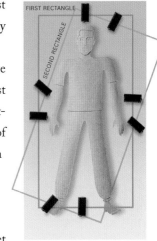

ABOVE *This layout uses tourmaline crystals, which attune the physical body to the planetary energies as a whole.*

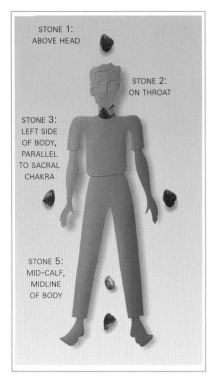

ETHERIC BODY LAYOUT

Etheric Body Layout

Giving healing energy to the etheric body will greatly accelerate the repair of physical tissues and may prevent other imbalances from gravitating into the physical body. Any period of illness or recuperation would benefit from this layout.

Six carnelians are needed. One is placed at the throat and one above the top of the head. At the level of the sacral chakra, a carnelian is placed on each side of the body. The remaining two stones are put on the midline of the body, one between the legs at about midcalf level and the last stone near the ankles. An orange-colored background to lie on will accentuate this layout's healing potential. Orange, the color of the sacral chakra, is the ideal vibration for repairing shock to the system.

Emotional Body Layout

The emotional body is the next vibratory level beyond the etheric. The etheric body holds the pattern for the physical body, and the emotional body contains the volatile and changing energy of our moods.

Visiting somewhere beautiful can change how we feel quite dramatically, but the opposite is also true. A beautiful scene can mean nothing to us if we are in a bad mood. The same street can be threatening and dangerous if we have just lost our money or the happiest if we have fallen in love. Music can provoke the deepest-felt emotions almost against our will or better judgment. A color, scent, or word can provoke intense irritation or melt our hearts. Emotion is the weather within us. It comes and goes, changes and flows continually. It hardly seems trustworthy or stable enough to base any decision on emotion,

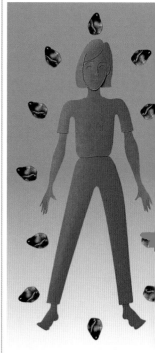

EMOTIONAL BODY LAYOUT

and yet, with most people, no matter how rationally important issues may be considered, the final choice is frequently made by following an emotional preference.

Emotions can play a huge part in our health and well-being. Emotional balance is not an unfeeling, neutral state, but a center point to which the system can return between extremes of happiness and sorrow. Without this balance or axis as a natural resting place, the emotions can get stuck in a way that is inappropriate and deleterious to the whole body. Holding onto a particular sort of emotional energy disrupts the whole body weather system. Damaging emotional storms and unseasonal climate can create profoundly unhealthy conditions for the individual.

For balancing and healing the emotional body, 12 smoky quartz crystals with their points directed outward are evenly spread around the body. The simplest way of doing this is to place one stone at the top of the head and one below the feet, then space five crystals evenly on each side of the body. An orange-colored background will accentuate the cleansing, flowing, and stabilizing qualities of the stones.

This emotional body layout is useful for increasing the healing potential of the body. It will also help reduce the effects of both trauma and stress.

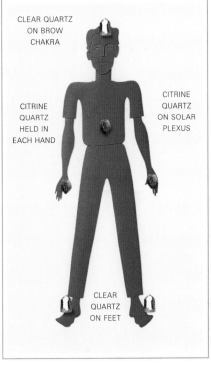

MENTAL BODY LAYOUT

Mental Body Layout

Since our emotions are translated into thoughts and we seem to respond to most stimuli emotionally, it can be difficult to define the difference between the mind and the emotions. The mental body, however, does have distinct and discrete properties. The emotional body reacts; the mental body records, categorizes, and files these reactions. The mental body, from birth, constructs how we perceive the world and the way it seems to work. The mental body creates our core beliefs and then attaches all other experiences around these central truths. Because these structures are so fundamental to our sense of ourselves, they can be difficult for us to see.

Core beliefs can exist in complete contradiction to each other, so, when a certain issue arises, these conflicts can create great stress. This stress very often translates into muscular tension and physical rigidity. Easing mental body issues can allow relaxation at many different levels, from posture to tolerance of others' beliefs, to flexibility in problem solving and finding positive options.

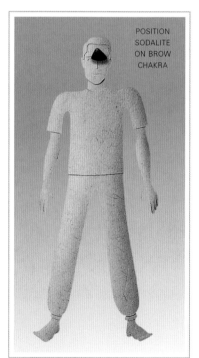

The layout that helps balance the mental body will also tend to improve all types of communication skills, speed of thought, clarity of mind, and coordination. A citrine quartz is held in each hand with its point facing down and away from the body. A third citrine is placed at the solar plexus, also point down. This stone will help activate the central nervous system, while the hand-held stones balance brain function. Clear quartz crystals are taped onto the top of each foot between the second and third toes, again pointing down, helping anchor the mental energy into practical areas of life.

POSITION SODALITE ON BROW CHAKRA

CAUSAL BODY LAYOUT

A clear quartz is placed on the forehead, pointing up toward the top of the head, energizing the brow chakra's perceptive abilities, enabling it to re-examine old truths in the light of greater understanding.

Causal Body Layout

To balance the causal body, which can be seen as the projector that puts our image onto the screen of physical existence, lie on a blue-colored cloth and then place a sodalite stone on the brow chakra at the center of your forehead.

Astral Body Layout

Within the astral body are all aspects of the individual personality. It is the container that allows us to recognize ourselves as unique beings. The astral body filters and tones down all other sources of energy and information so as not to overwhelm individual consciousness. Weakness at this level can create great confusion in our perception of reality. Too closed an astral body prevents useful information or other dimensions of energy from integrating into everyday consciousness, leading to feelings of isolation and loss of direction.

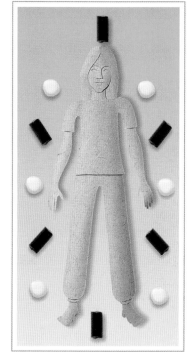

ASTRAL BODY LAYOUT

This layout is enhanced when laid out on a cloth of deep pink or magenta. This helps access the underlying universal flows of energy. Twelve crystals are used in this layout—six tumbled pieces of milky quartz and six of black tourmaline. Milky quartz is a translucent white variety commonly found among river and seashore pebbles. The pebble form accentuates the gentle expansive sphere of protective energy emanating from this stone. The black tourmaline anchors the energy of the self; together, these stones can balance the polarities implicit in the functions of the astral body. Put one tourmaline above the head, one below the feet, and alternate the remaining quartz and tourmalines evenly around the body.

The finer levels of the subtle anatomy can be both accessed and positively altered by crystal healing.

Soul Body Layout

The soul, or celestial body, the sixth subtle energy envelope that interpenetrates all the other levels, including the physical, can be brought into greater balance with seven small clusters of celestite. Celestite, or celestine, is a beautiful pale blue mineral that forms clusters of soft heavy crystals. It is wonderful for lifting dark moods and bringing a subtle bliss to perceptions. Only small clusters of celestite crystals are needed, but it may take some hunting to find suitable pieces. Most people find this layout enjoyable, although it often requires considerable grounding afterward.

A white cloth will amplify the ethereal effects of the stones, which should be placed as follows: one cluster above the head, one beside each shoulder, one at the side of each thigh, and one beside each ankle, if possible facing toward the body. With this layout, it is easier to attune to fine levels of inspiration. There can be relief from worldly pressures and a sense of spiritual uplift, fulfillment, and cleansing.

Spiritual Body Layout

The finest level of which we are aware, the spiritual body, encompasses our whole existence in and outside of time and space, so no single method is likely to bring balance to the whole.

This layout helps bring conscious awareness to the multidimensional reality and timeless nature of the self. It can access information from the very deepest levels of consciousness and from different parts of the universe, helping to integrate knowledge of our true direction and increasing our overall sense of purpose. Often this profound information will take the form of dreams, ideas, or inspiration.

This layout is best done on a white cloth and needs three clear quartz, four amethyst, and five pieces of moldavite. Large pieces can be expensive, but small fragments will work just as well.

Moldavite is put in both hands, on the center of the forehead, and taped on top of each foot between the first and second toes. The clear quartz makes a triangle, one piece on each side of the body, about level with the solar plexus, and one below the feet, all with points inward. The four amethysts form a rectangle around the body: two above the head about shoulder-width apart, and one on each side of the legs just below the knees.

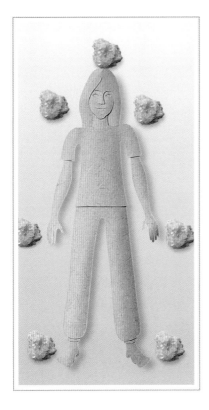

RIGHT *Clusters of celestite bring relief from worldly concerns.*

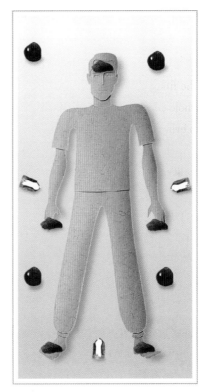

LEFT *The spiritual body layout increases self-confidence and helps us focus our energies in a meaningful direction.*

SUBTLE BODIES STONE PLACEMENT

Use an assessment technique, such as dowsing or muscle testing, to find out which subtle bodies could benefit from this process. Place the stones in their correct locations and check how long they need to remain in place. After removing the stones, recheck the subtle bodies to see that all of them have been balanced.

BODY	FOCUS/PLACEMENT OF STONES	BALANCING STONES
ETHERIC BODY	No specified points of focus, since the etheric body is completely interconnected with the physical. Find out—for example, by dowsing—where the stones should be placed.	Abalone, azurite, amazonite, azurite, malachite, aventurine, aquamarine, bloodstone, chrysoprase, fluorite, clear quartz, galena, Herkimer diamond, garnet, picture jasper, jet, kunzite, jade, green jasper, lapis lazuli, lodestone, malachite, topaz.
EMOTIONAL BODY	Stomach	Botswana agate, fire agate, moss agate, serpentine, aventurine, azurite, malachite, emerald, Herkimer diamond, jade, meteorite, sphene, green jasper, jet, moonstone, obsidian, opal, amethyst, smoky quartz, citrine, rose quartz, clear quartz, rhyolite, sapphire.
MENTAL BODY	Left hemisphere of the brain. Place the stone or stones around the left side of the head. Check the correct position for each.	Fire agate, moss agate, amazonite, amber, aquamarine, aventurine, azurite, green jasper, diamond, gold, lapis lazuli, meteorite, morganite, obsidian, dark opal, amethyst, smoky quartz, citrine, rose quartz, clear quartz, ruby, sphene.

SUBTLE BODIES STONE PLACEMENT (CONTINUED)

BODY	FOCUS/PLACEMENT OF STONES	BALANCING STONES
ASTRAL BODY	Kidneys. Check to see if different stones are needed near each kidney or whether the same one is needed on both sides of the body. Tuck the appropriate stones under the back at about the level of the elbow.	Copper, emerald, Herkimer diamond, jade, green jasper, meteorite, moonstone, peridot, iron pyrites, smoky quartz, citrine, rose quartz, rhodochrosite, sapphire, serpentine, silver.
CAUSAL BODY	Medulla oblongata at the base of the skull.	No specific selection of stone is suggested. You will need to determine the most appropriate stone in each case.
SOUL BODY	Pineal gland. The easiest placement here is at the center of the forehead.	Citrine quartz.
SPIRITUAL BODY	Pituitary gland. Test for the best placement, which might be beside the head, level with the ears, behind the crown, or at the forehead.	Sphene, ruby, citrine, amethyst, lapis lazuli, gold, garnet, carnelian.

Cleansing the Aura

*I*f the aura needs cleansing, this can he done by placing stones on appropriate spots or by sweeping stones through the aura, either held in the hand or on a pendulum.

The Cleansing Process

Use a method such as dowsing or muscle testing to assess which subtle bodies would benefit from balance of the auric field.

Once the general picture is clear, identify the appropriate stones you are to use for each subtle body. Choose from sapphire, ruby, smoky quartz, lodestone, green jasper, or Herkimer diamond, but always check to see if something else is needed since there may be an ideal stone not listed here. Several stones may be needed for each placement. Every crystal healing session deals with the unique energies of an individual. Techniques offer useful guidelines but are flexible. You should always check to see whether there is anything else required.

RIGHT *Together with lodestone and green jasper, these stones are ideal for aura cleansing. Draw each stone through the aura or place them on or around the body.*

RUBY

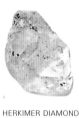

HERKIMER DIAMOND

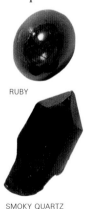

SMOKY QUARTZ

SAPPHIRE

Place the stone or stones in the identified area, check that it is correct, and the length of time they are to be left in place. When checking how long the stones should be left, wait until all the stones are in position. It may have taken you several minutes to complete each layout so that some stones will have been in place quite a long time before the question is asked. The question can be framed: "How much longer do the stones...?"

It may be that the stones will need to be removed in a particular order. Check beforehand. When they are removed, recheck the subtle bodies for balance.

Complete the balance by sweeping the aura with your hands, thereby normalizing the energy levels and stabilizing the correction.

CONSTRUCTION OF AN AURAMETER

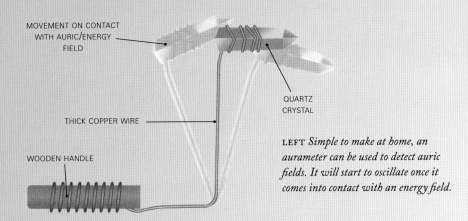

MOVEMENT ON CONTACT WITH AURIC/ENERGY FIELD

QUARTZ CRYSTAL

THICK COPPER WIRE

WOODEN HANDLE

LEFT *Simple to make at home, an aurameter can be used to detect auric fields. It will start to oscillate once it comes into contact with an energy field.*

Additional Practice

When you can quickly identify another person's auric field, see if you can isolate its different layers, mental, emotional, astral, and so on. Approach the subject slowly, from some distance. Don't be surprised if the auric fields appear to extend farther than you had expected.

This exercise can also be done using a pendulum or by self-testing. An aurameter *(see box on page 163)* is a specialized pendulum that is used to register auric fields. One can be made easily by wrapping thick copper wire around a quartz crystal and then attaching the free end to a handle of some kind. Put a right-angle bend in the wire, and it will indicate by a clear horizontal oscillation when it encounters an energy field.

Try the following exercise. Have someone you know stand up just a short distance from you, so that it is easy for you to scan the whole body. Now swiftly look to feel or sense their aura. If it helps, make a simple sketch and note down any areas that feel different. First, look or feel what the aura is like as a whole. Is it balanced? Or is it top or bottom-heavy? Does it feel as though it extends evenly around the physical body, or are there variations? Is your attention drawn to particular areas, and, if so, how do they feel? Try to describe these sensations in sense words: tactile, aural, or visual.

Practice this sensing with friends and strangers. Remember not to focus too hard or to concentrate or intellectualize the process. This relaxed, neutral, aura scanning technique can prove valuable for identifying areas needing attention.

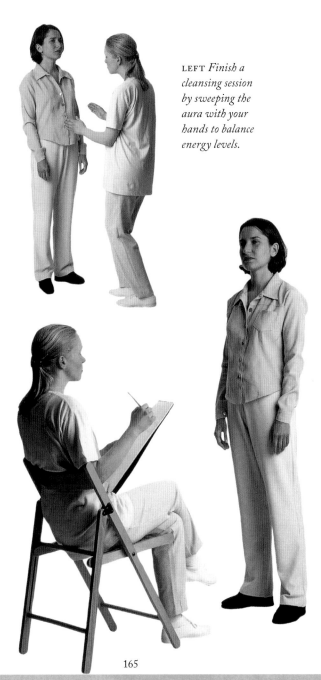

LEFT *Finish a cleansing session by sweeping the aura with your hands to balance energy levels.*

LEFT *Practice aura reading on a friend. It may help to sketch out what you sense in each area.*

The Meridian System

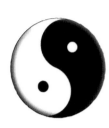

ABOVE *Yin and yang represent opposing, yet interdependent, energies in all things.*

*T*he meridian system of subtle energy is at the heart of traditional Chinese medicine. Knowledge of the meridians and the acupuncture points requires extensive in-depth study. Because of this, most crystal healers rarely work with the meridian system. There are, however, useful healing procedures that combine the energy of crystals with meridian energies in straightforward ways. Once there is confidence in an assessment technique, such as dowsing or muscle testing, the correct placement of a specific stone on a meridian point can make dramatic changes to a person's well-being.

The meridian system, as conceived by the Chinese, has 12 main energy channels that follow recognized pathways near the surface of the skin. Although it is one integrated system, each meridian has a starting point and an end point, which indicates direction of flow and function. Each meridian is named after an organ or function, such as the liver or stomach, but this can be misleading in the West, as the physical organ is only a small aspect of the type of energy with which a meridian deals. The functions ascribed to physical organs by the Chinese rarely have any recognizable Western correlations.

It has been generally thought that the meridians are nonphysical, or etheric, vessels providing the physical body with the subtle nutrition of chi, or life energy. Recent research suggests that meridians are, at least at some levels, superfine, physical structures. The acupuncture points along each meridian have been clearly identified as having a different electrical potential to non-acupuncture points. Injecting minute amounts of a marker substance has demonstrated that it migrates rapidly out from the acupressure point along very specific pathways distinct from any nerve or blood vessels. Close examination of these pathways shows a system that parallels and interweaves with known physical organs and systems. It contains a fluid that has some similarities to blood and lymph. When experimenters severed these channels around an organ, cellular disruption followed. The arrangement of this microscopic system suggests that it comes into being before any other cellular differentiation and may act as a template for the development of the body.

In addition to the 12 meridians that flow on each side of the body, there are many other vessels that feed the chi energy into smaller channels for distribution. The most important extra channels are the Conception Vessel and Governing Vessel, both of which possess acupuncture points and flow up the midline of the body. These two channels help maintain the flow of chi within the entire system and affect vitality and health.

Meridian Balancing with a Quartz

Hold the center of a double-terminateed clear quartz between the thumb and index finger and turn it around with the other hand for about a minute. This process is then repeated with all the other fingers, using the thumb as the balance point. Repeat the procedure with the other hand.

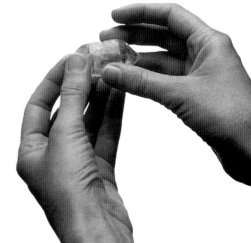

RIGHT *Roll a clear quartz crystal between each finger and the thumb in turn. This balances the meridians.*

THE MERIDIANS AND THEIR EMOTIONAL CONNOTATIONS

One simple way of understanding some of the functions of the meridians is to associate them with emotional states. Thus, a positive emotion will energize or strengthen a meridian, while its corresponding negative emotional expression will tend to reduce the energy or weaken the meridian. In this way, it is possible to identify some of the underlying emotional energy causing disruption to the system. John Diamond, a pioneering kinesiologist, has discovered the attributes of the meridians and emotional states.

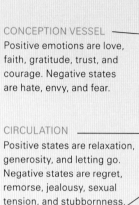

FRONT

BACK

CONCEPTION VESSEL
Positive emotions are love, faith, gratitude, trust, and courage. Negative states are hate, envy, and fear.

CIRCULATION
Positive states are relaxation, generosity, and letting go. Negative states are regret, remorse, jealousy, sexual tension, and stubbornness.

HEART
Positive emotions are love and forgiveness. Negative emotion is anger.

SPLEEN
Positive emotions are faith, security, and confidence about the future. Negative emotions are realistic anxieties about the future.

STOMACH
Positive emotions are contentment and tranquility. Negative states are disappointment, disgust, bitterness, greed, nausea, hunger, and emptiness.

GALL BLADDER
Positive emotions are reaching out with love, forgiveness, and adoration. Negative emotions are rage, fury, and wrath.

KIDNEY
Positive states relate to sexual assuredness. Negative states relate to sexual indecision.

LUNG
Positive emotions are humility, tolerance, and modesty. Negative states are disdain, contempt, and prejudice.

LIVER
Positive emotions are happiness. Negative emotions are misery, woe, and sadness.

GOVERNING VESSEL
There are no specific emotional states listed except as for the central meridian, the Conception Vessel.

BLADDER
Positive emotions are peace. Negative emotions are restlessness and frustration.

TRIPLE WARMER
Positive emotions are elation, hope, lightness and buoyancy. Negative states are loneliness, despondency, grief, hopelessness, despair and depression.

LARGE INTESTINE (COLON)
Positive emotions are self-worth and acceptance. Negative state is guilt.

SMALL INTESTINE
Positive state is joy. Negative states are sadness and sorrow.

ABOVE AND RIGHT *The 12 main meridians of traditional Chinese medicine are paired on each side of the body. The two central channels, the Conception and Governing vessels, influence the yin and yang meridians respectively.*

Meridian Massage

*M*eridian massage helps balance the whole meridian system by reinforcing the natural direction of each meridian's flow. The flow of energy around the body often becomes sluggish or reversed when the body and mind have been placed under long-term stress or immediate shock. Although it is a simple technique, meridian massage can have profound beneficial effects and makes a calming and highly therapeutic daily practice.

SELF-MASSAGE PROCEDURE

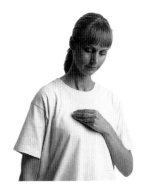

1 *Choose an appropriate stone, by dowsing if necessary. With the stone in your left hand, starting at the heart, move up along the chest and down the inside of the right arm.*

2 *Move around the fingers and up the outside of the arm to the shoulder and neck.*

3 *Repeat the movement with the stone in your right hand on your left side.*

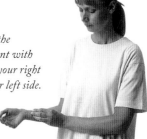

MOVE STONE
DOWN THE ARMS

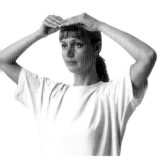

4 *With both hands together, sweep up your face and over your head as far down the neck and back as you can go.*

5 *Then reach up your back and sweep the crystal down your back and down the backs of your legs to your feet.*

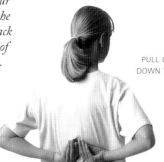

PULL CRYSTAL
DOWN THE BACK

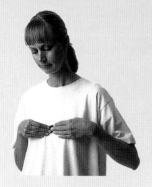

DRAW STONE
FROM BASE
CHAKRA TO LIP

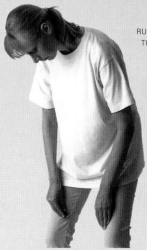

RUN CRYSTAL UP
THE INSIDE OF
THE LEG

6 *Pass around your feet and back up the inside of your legs and midline to your heart. This is one circuit.*

7 *After finishing a number of circuits, move the stone from the base chakra to the lower lip several times.*

8 *Then move the stone or crystal from the base of the spine and up the backbone as far as possible and then reach over your head to draw the crystal across your upper back, head, and face to your upper lip. Repeat this movement several times.*

GIVING A MASSAGE

Stand in front of the patient and keep your hands 1 to 2 inches (2–5 cm) away from the body throughout the massage.

1 *Ask the person to stand comfortably, with legs slightly apart and arms held away from the body, palms facing toward the body.*

2 *Choose two appropriate crystals or tumbled stones. Each stone should be large enough to cover the palm of your hand.*

3 *Holding a crystal in each hand, begin with both hands over the heart area.*

4 *Sweep up to the armpits and along the insides of the arms to the hands.*

5 *Pass over the fingers and return up the outsides of the arms to the shoulders, meeting again at the throat.*

6 *Sweep both crystals up the face and over the head, following as closely as possible down the midline of the back and then down the backs of the legs to the feet. You might not be able to fully reach around the person's back. This is not too important. Anywhere that you have to leave the exact line, simply use the intention of your mind to complete the sweep across the appropriate area.*

7 Pass around the toes and up the inside of the legs and then on up the midline of the torso to the heart. This is one circuit. The number of circuits and the speed at which you move is up to you.

8 Move to one side and complete the sweep up the Conception and Governing vessels by simultaneously passing both stones up the front and back midlines from the base to the lips.

9 Repeat several times. Sometimes it may be better to hold a different sort of stone in each hand. If this is the case, check to see if you need to swap them after a number of circuits to balance the stones' energies.

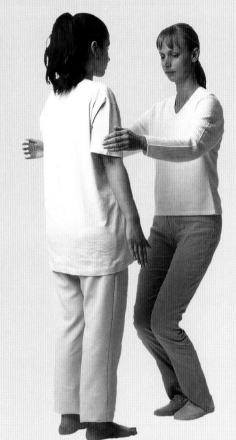

LEFT *Sweep the crystals from the person's hands and up the arms to the shoulders and onto the throat.*

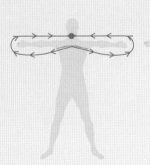
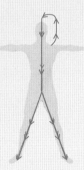
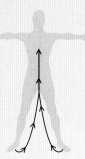

FRONT   BACK   FRONT

LEFT *Complete a full circuit of the body according to the routes shown. Repeat the procedure as many times as you wish.*

Crystals and the Meridian System

A balanced meridian system usually means that there is neither a lack of energy nor an excess of energy in the system. Individual meridians or parts of meridians may be working outside their normal ranges, but in a balanced system the general equilibrium is kept by an excess in one area being balanced by a lack in another. Sometimes a localized imbalance needs to be corrected to bring about healing.

REBALANCING A MERIDIAN

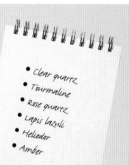

- Clear quartz
- Tourmaline
- Rose quartz
- Lapis lazuli
- Heliodor
- Amber

1 To determine which meridians need balancing, use an arc or list to dowse or do a muscle test. Remember that apart from the Conception and Governing vessels, all meridians are in pairs.

2 Determine which side of the meridian pair needs balancing or whether both sides require attention.

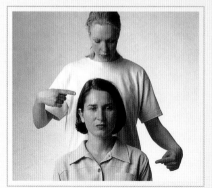

3 An effective demonstration of an imbalanced meridian can be to lightly touch one end point with a couple of fingers. If that half of the meridian is out of balance, a previously strong muscle test will go weak. Muscle testing all meridians in this way, called "therapy localizing," will quickly show where work is needed.

4 In this method, it is not important which end point is touched, so choose whichever is most convenient. The point can be held by either the tester or the patient.

5 Once all meridians have been tested, find out which crystals will rebalance them. If you are dowsing, then work by color categories or lists. If you are muscle testing, start in the same way with color categories.

6 Once the stone is identified, ask on which end point it needs to be placed and for how long. You will probably need to tape the stone in place.

7 Check to see if stones are needed at one end only or both ends of the meridian.

8 *If stones are needed at both ends of the meridian, find whether different sorts of stones are necessary.*

9 *Once the process is completed and the stones removed, recheck all the meridians to make sure everything is in balance. If you are muscle testing, localize each point after the crystals have been removed to check on the efficacy of the rebalancing.*

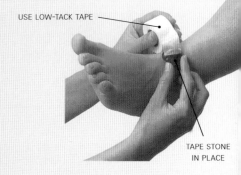

USE LOW-TACK TAPE

TAPE STONE IN PLACE

EFFECTS OF REBALANCING

▲ Like every other subtle system, and even the body's physical systems, a small change in one area may create a large effect overall. It is not possible to isolate one part from the whole. This means that care must always be taken to carry out only appropriate healing work.

▲ Sometimes the correction is at such a deep level that nothing much is experienced immediately. On the other hand, this technique can initiate some strange subjective feelings and emotions.

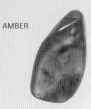

AMBER

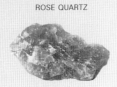

ROSE QUARTZ

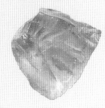

HELIODOR

Acupuncture Point Corrections

The meridian system may appear balanced even when individual acupuncture points may be seriously overenergized or underenergized, and occasionally it is necessary and appropriate to work with single points rather than end points. This is usually very powerful, and care needs to be taken to make sure the body has plenty of time to readjust and assimilate the changes. A rest period of several weeks, free of any other healing work, is usual.

ACUPRESSURE POINT PROCEDURE

1 *Determine that it is appropriate and safe to work with an acupressure point by dowsing or muscle testing.*

2 *Find which meridian is involved, using dowsing or muscle testing.*

3 *Find out whether the left or right channels need work.*

4 *Find the exact spot to place the stone by lightly tracing the path of the meridian with your fingertips until your arm or pendulum indicates the correct spot. Always start from the beginning of the meridian and work toward the end. This way, you will be prevented from inadvertently weakening the meridian by moving against the flow.*

5 *Mark the correct spot with a piece of tape.*

6 *Work out the type of crystal needed and how long it needs to be in place. Don't put the stone on the point until you have all the information that you require.*

7 *When placing the stone, double-check the exact location.*

8 *Monitor carefully how the patient feels during the period of placement.*

9 *When the correction is complete, remove the stone and retest to check that all is okay.*

10 *Make sure the patient is fully grounded and suggest they drink a little more water than usual for a few days to help the internal cleansing process.*

Sometimes an exact stone is needed, so if you have several pieces of the indicated crystal, test each one to find the best one possible for your subject. It is not necessary to know the exact point required if the meridian is traced. If you have a diagram of the acupressure points, identify the necessary place and then check the exact location on the body. It may differ slightly from the diagram.

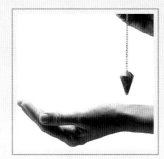

ABOVE *Dowse the acupressure point to find out whether it is a suitable area in which to work.*

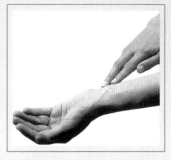

ABOVE *Run your fingers lightly along the meridian to determine where the stone should be placed.*

Figure-eight Circuits

*I*n Tibetan healing systems, there are a series of energy channels in the body that can be simplified as figure-eight patterns. Each of these circuits always flows in the same direction, but where there is stress or a blockage of energy, it may start moving in the opposite way, depriving the body of an important energy source.

SCHORL

SMOKY QUARTZ

CLEAR QUARTZ

The Circuits

One set of circuits is located on the front of the body, and a corresponding set is on the back. Front and back, there are a total of six figure-eights to check.

• A lower circuit moves between the hips and the feet.
• A middle circuit exists on the abdomen between the shoulders and the pelvis.
• An upper circuit lies between the top of the head and the neck.

Where there is felt to be a significant area of unmoving or stagnant energy in the subtle systems, or when there is a need to shift a buildup of stress out of the aura, or when there seems to be a general lack of integration between the upper and lower halves of the body, perhaps manifesting as a lack of coordination or being grounded, it might be appropriate to create a figure-eight pattern around the whole body.

• First, check the whole body circuit. If dowsing with a pendulum, ask if it is balanced and strong.
• If weak, check in which direction the flow needs to move to restrengthen it.
• Correct this circuit first, but if it tests okay, check the six smaller circuits for imbalances.

ABOVE *Smoky quartz and schorl are the most fitting for this procedure; clear quartz is an alternative.*

A circuit can be rebalanced by making a figure-eight with crystals of smoky quartz or black tourmaline, which are both ideal cleansers and removers of imbalance from many levels, physical and subtle. If your crystals have natural terminations, place them in the direction of flow. If you have no terminated stones or only tumbled stones, use a larger single quartz crystal and sweep it over the stones in the required direction several times.

If you are muscle testing for assessment, a downward pass from shoulder to the opposite hip will weaken a strong indicator muscle if the circuit needs strengthening. In this case, the stones are pointed in the direction where a pass from shoulder to hip or hip to shoulder remains strong. The correction has been successful when, on retesting, passes in all directions stay strong.

The crystals can be placed on or off the body, and you might need some tape to keep some in place. The number of crystals you use is less important than their positions and direction, but try to keep a balanced, symmetrical placement.

Figure-eight energies can be corrected by using a single, large crystal. Slowly and purposefully direct the crystal point down toward the body, along the path of the circuit. Repeat the loops until the energy returns to normal levels.

Sometimes there is a need to revitalize an area of the body to remove stress or tension. Here, a figure-eight might be useful, especially if there appears to be a lack of integration with the body as a whole. This can often be the case with longstanding or particularly unpleasant ailments. In these situations, the figure-eights may be needed in a very particular part of the body different from the circuits already covered here. Many other smaller circuits also exist—for example, along the arms or in the feet, which may need stimulating.

FIGURE-EIGHT CIRCUITS

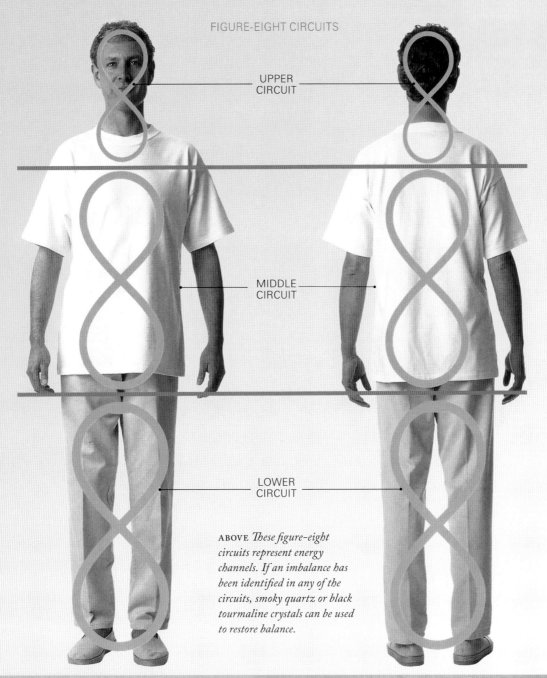

UPPER
CIRCUIT

MIDDLE
CIRCUIT

LOWER
CIRCUIT

ABOVE *These figure–eight circuits represent energy channels. If an imbalance has been identified in any of the circuits, smoky quartz or black tourmaline crystals can be used to restore balance.*

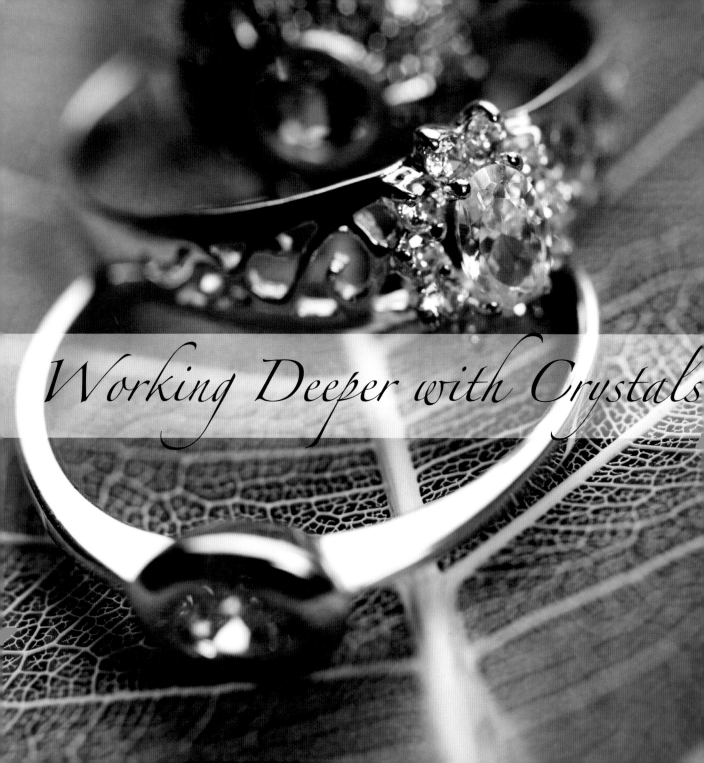

Working Deeper with Crystals

Hand-held Crystals

Many crystal healers use a single large clear quartz to energize or cleanse the auric field. Intention and visualization are an important part of the effectiveness of this method, and like all other processes in which the healer becomes actively involved, special care must be given to grounding and centering at all times—before, during, and after the session.

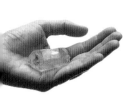

ABOVE *Holding a large, clear quartz crystal in your hand can stimulate or cleanse the aura.*

Whenever we think of someone we know, a natural resonance is created. When we wish someone well, there is an automatic flow of healing energy, and this energy can easily be concentrated and enhanced with quartz crystals.

A stunning demonstration of how sensitive each one of us is to the thoughts of others uses muscle testing. A strong muscle will weakens dramatically if the subject is the focus of a negative thought. Conversely, a weak muscle will strengthen with a positive, life-affirming thought. This is a clear illustration of the fact that those in healing situations need to cultivate positive values, not artificial moods, and should be personally committed to continuing self-development.

The first thing to establish is what methods feel right for you personally. If a recommended process doesn't feel comfortable, it will not be fully effective because, in these situations, it is the mind that directs and controls the flow of healing energy.

Working with hand-held crystals differs from the laying of stones in that the healer is more energetically involved in the healing process. Whatever technique is used, even absent healing creates an immediate link between healer and patient. This cannot be avoided. There is, however, a difference in degree of emotional and empathic response. To make sure that only appropriate work is done, it is necessary to remain truly grounded and centered and to be fully aware of how the patient is feeling during the process.

The body has a natural polarity, and various parts act like the north and south poles of a magnet. Usually, opposite sides of the body have opposite polarity. If opposite polarities are brought together, there tends to be a flow of life energy between them. Generally speaking, the right hand is positively charged in right-handed people, and the left hand is positively charged in left-handed people.

Finding Your Own Energy Flow

The positively charged hand always radiates, or gives out energy, while the negatively charged hand tends to absorb and receive energy.

This simple exercise helps establish which is your energizing, and which your healing, hand.

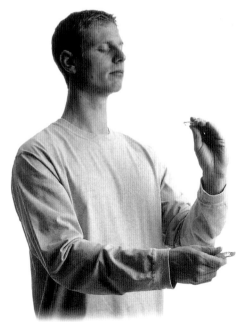

BELOW *Use two quartz crystals to experience your energy field and to find out which way it flows.*

1. Hold a quartz crystal in your left palm pointed in and another crystal in your right palm, pointed out.

2. Imagine a flow of energy going through your body between these points from the inward-pointing crystals to the outward-pointing crystal.

3. Now reverse the points of each stone and imagine the flow in the opposite direction.

The direction that feels the most comfortable is your natural flow from receiving (negative, yin) to energizing (positive, yang).

This natural flow of energy can be directed and amplified by holding a crystal in one or the other hand.

A crystal tends to focus energy in the direction in which its point is facing. By changing the position of a crystal and the hand in which it is held, a crystal healer can control flows of energy in the body. The two main processes of hand-held crystal healing are to release and clear areas of excess energy and to energize areas with a lack of energy, or under energy.

Clearing Over Energy

Areas of over energy are often indicated by feelings of tension, heat, pain, or congestion. Irritation, frustration, and anger may also be present. To clear this buildup of trapped energy, place your receiving hand palm down on the troubled area. In your energizing or directing hand, hold a clear quartz crystal with its point away from your body, facing down toward the ground.

Breathing deeply and evenly, imagine all the excess energy passing through your body via the receiving hand and out through the crystal in a more harmonious, balanced form and entering the Earth.

ABOVE *To recharge energy, hold the quartz in your energizing hand and point it toward the body. Cup a small stone in your receiving hand.*

Energizing the Body

An area that is low in energy feels heavy, sluggish, cold, and dull. There may be a general lack of enthusiasm or simply a feeling of tiredness. An increase of energy needs to be directed into this area, so the quartz crystal is now held in the energizing, or charging, hand, pointing toward the body. The receiving hand is held away from the body, palm upward, and is imagined absorbing life energy from the universe, which passes into the crystal and then into the body.

Holding another stone, such as a small sphere or tumbled stone, in the receiving hand helps transform the moving energies to become more coherent and balanced. You can use this technique either by yourself or with other people.

Moving the crystal in a particular way may serve to speed up the healing process. A counterclockwise circle tends to draw out and remove imbalances, while a clockwise circle infuses energy into an area. Allow your intuition and your body's intelligence to direct you to move the crystal in an appropriate way.

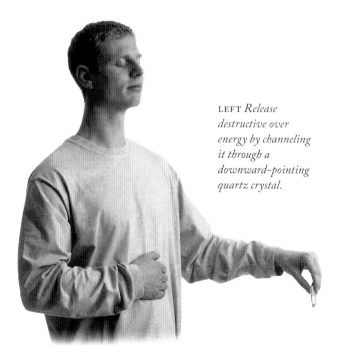

LEFT *Release destructive over energy by channeling it through a downward-pointing quartz crystal.*

Working with Two Crystals

*M*uch useful healing can be achieved with different combinations of hand-held stones and the conscious directing of energy using the imaginative and visualizing mind of the healer.

Using Two Crystal Points

• To increase the flow of energy through a blocked area (where there is nerve damage, for example), a crystal can be held on each side of the block with both points indicating the direction of flow. Tracing the line of the energy flow with one crystal point can also work well.

• Hold two points toward an area lacking in vitality and visualize a flow of life-supporting energy or light flowing through the crystals.

• To clear a small area, or one perceived as deep within the body, a crystal point can be directed downward to feed in positive healing energy. The second crystal, in the other hand, can be held point outward to draw out and cleanse the released stress.

The coherent organization of crystal lattices will always tend to increase the order of negatively perceived energies. If kept cleansed, a crystal will thus act as a transformer of disharmonious vibration.

Remember that imbalance, stress, and disease are simply the wrong sorts of energy in the wrong place. That energy, once removed from an aggravated situation, will not necessarily continue to cause a problem elsewhere. One person's inharmonious energy may be exactly what someone else lacks.

Using a Crystal Point and Sphere

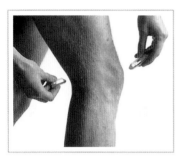

ABOVE *Crystals can help when held on either side of an area where there is poor blood flow, nerve damage, or scar tissue.*

• A crystal point naturally directs energy, while holding a smooth stone in front of the crystal point that diffuses the energy, will allow it to enter the aura in a gentler, smoother way. This same position can also be used to modify the quality of one crystal with another. For example, the frictionless clarity of selenite can be slowed and diffused by placing a moonstone sphere, egg, or tumbled stone in the path of its energy stream. The energies of one stone are focused through the lens of another and are diffused by the rounded shape into a patient's aura.

• It is also possible to channel, focus, and draw the energy qualities of the sphere through a pointed crystal. A clear quartz can absorb and direct the healing characteristics of another stone. Using a sequence of tumbled stones at the same point can feed a variety of energies into the aura.

• Where healing in an area is required, a sphere or egg can be gently moved through the auric field diffusing positive energy, while the point can be directed to remove and transform energy debris outward.

• The point can be used like a wand to cut or loosen blocks, while the sphere smooths and reseals the healed areas.

RIGHT *In this way of working, crystals are seen as channels, conduits, or pipes for energy.*

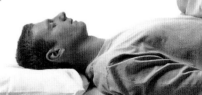

184

Record Keepers

Record-keeper crystals can reveal the history of the universe on physical and other dimensions. They are identified by perfect triangles etched or raised on one or more facets. They are said to be special crystals within which wisdom has been stored consciously by other beings. The triangular formations may allow clearer access to information present in many, if not all, crystals.

Procedure for Record Keepers

1. Closely examine the crystal and especially the record-keeper's triangle. Hold the shape in mind.

2. Close your eyes, quietening your breathing, perhaps repeat a mantra or say "Om" a few times to help your awareness settle down.

3. Imagine the crystal in front of you and the triangular mark of the record keeper on your forehead.

4. See the crystal increasing in size until it is much larger than you.

5. Imagine you are moving closer to the crystal and be aware that you are looking for an entrance point. You may find yourself floating above or around the faces of the stone as if you were on an invisible escalator.

6. It is likely that there will be some kind of triangular door. Move over to the door and place your forehead against its surface.

7. If you are allowed or are ready, you will find yourself inside the energy form of the crystal and will be able to receive information that will be of use to you.

8. When this process is over, or you wish to leave, return to the door, place your forehead with its triangular mark to the door once more, and find yourself outside the crystal.

9. Move away from the crystal and become gradually aware of your body. Thank the crystal's energies and will it to return to its physical size.

10. Take time to record and assess the experiences you have had.

11. Visit the record-keeper's crystal form often to attune your energies and to deepen the whole experience.

Many people consider the etched markings of some crystals to indicate particular history or information within the stone. Maybe the evocative symbols and hieroglyphic-type markings can put us in touch with more universal aspects of the self, freeing us to experience levels of awareness and information not usually available to the conscious mind. If you have a crystal whose markings you find fascinating, carry out the above exercise while visualizing the particular shapes instead of the triangular door. Contemporary society frequently sees coincidences, objects, and events as materialistic things rather than as symbols of a deeper reality. This view might free us from the fear of powerful spirits, but it increases our profound sense of isolation and can be psychologically damaging. Using the patterns, veils, etchings, and shapes of crystals to free the mind from its everyday constraints and organization can lead to an increase in well-being and a clearer view of reality.

Whether an experience is worthwhile and valid depends not upon how objectively real it might be, but on how much it improves one's enjoyment of life and sense of well-being.

BELOW *Imagine the imprint of the crystal on your forehead and let it send information into your mind.*

Programming Crystals

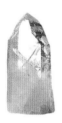

*T*he process of programming a crystal, so that the energy structures within the atomic lattice are modified, focuses the activity and energy of the crystal toward specific desired goals. Crystals can be programmed by the active method, which uses the projection of conscious thought energy. The passive method works by repeated use.

Programming a crystal will amplify whatever intent is placed within it so that it reflects back on the subtle levels of awareness. However, as a neutral mirror, without any participation of its own spirit or awareness, a programmed crystal can be a devastating tool if misused.

Whether an active or passive programming method is used, that vibration of energy has to be in harmony with the crystal's own energy in order for it to work in a positive, life-enhancing way for both you and the crystal. As with all crystal work, it is important to remember that it is a joint effort between you and the stone.

Passive programming is easier to do, and, by its very nature, it is a less intrusive method. It works by orienting the main energy of a crystal in a certain way. Using exposure over time, to a distinct and coherent external influence, such as color, particular sound, favorite scent, symbol, and so on, that specific energy pattern is held within the memory—the energetic structures of the matrix. Thus a clear quartz that has been passively programmed with blue light will work as clear quartz, but in a blue sort of way.

IDEAS FOR PROGRAMS

Any crystal will be able to accept programming. However, clear quartz is the favored stone simply because it has a broad range of functions and is more or less neutral. This enables quartz to work easily with a wider range of situations than most other crystals.

• A frequent suggestion is that newly acquired crystals can be programmed so that they remain free of negative influences or can only be used for life-supporting ends. While these are noble sentiments, in almost all cases, the crystal structure itself will deal with most energy imbalances and will work to increase harmony and coherence. On the other hand, if a piece of crystal jewelry is worn often, it could be programmed to become more efficient at self-cleansing. Jewelry can also be programmed to enhance specific qualities, such as confidence, clarity of mind, protection from harm, health, and so on.

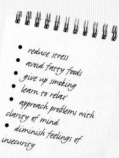

RIGHT *Think about areas of your life where crystals could exert a benevolent influence.*

- reduce stress
- avoid fatty foods
- give up smoking
- learn to relax
- approach problems with clarity of mind
- diminish feelings of insecurity

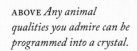

ABOVE *Any animal qualities you admire can be programmed into a crystal.*

• Where crystals are used for very particular purposes, whether programmed initially or not, they will become more and more effective so long as they are regularly checked to see if they need cleansing.

• If you learn to listen to each crystal's wishes, you will never have a shortage of ideas for programming.

• Choosing the exact nature of a program does need careful consideration. The more precise and detailed the wording of the intent, the greater its effectiveness will be. Programming a crystal for world peace is expecting a little too much, but "peace around me" or "peace in this room" is fine. Likewise, the word "health" is very general, while "relief from headaches," "strengthening heart function," "reducing tension," and so on is more focused.

• Try listening to the crystal itself, to see where it would appreciate its energies being directed. You may be surprised at the exact wording that enters your awareness.

• A crystal can be programmed with a piece of music that will continually radiate its qualities into a space. Likewise, a type of environment can be programmed, such as a sunset on a long beach, a rainforest, even another galaxy. Use sounds, pictures, and other means to program a crystal. The energy of a favorite animal or plant, a spiritual teacher, or some other holy image can be programmed into an appropriate stone, to energize and protect a space or individual.

• Some makers of flower essences, vibrational remedies prepared from plants, use programmed crystals to absorb the vibrational characteristics of flowers, rather than having to pick them. The crystal is then put into spring water, which it charges with the plant's energy.

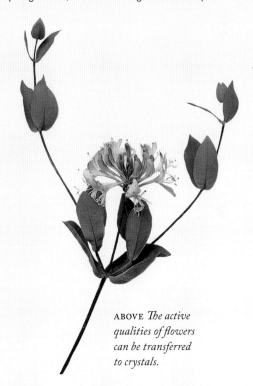

ABOVE *The active qualities of flowers can be transferred to crystals.*

Preliminaries

Attune to the crystal and decide whether you are completely happy with that crystal being modified, even if temporarily. Does it feel comfortable to work in this way with the crystal? Some crystals may have programs already or be working on a particular energy level. This must be checked beforehand.

1. Attune to the stone, using whichever exercises suit you best.

2. Ask permission of the crystal before you attempt programming.

3. Wait for a response. If it feels negative or there is doubt, you can attune further and ask again. If the feeling is still negative or doubtful, don't continue.

4. Ask the crystal to open a part of its matrix to accept the program.

5. Wait until you feel a new openness in the crystal's energy.

6. If you are to use the passive mode, put the crystal in the appropriate place and leave it for a while.

7. If you are using the active mode, work out the precise wording or the exact thought beforehand. Check and recheck its validity.

8. Allow the idea and the crystal to contact each other. Wait for a feeling of acceptance or resistance to the thought by floating the thought into the crystal.

9. If there is harmony, focus your awareness as closely as possible on the thought and project it into the crystal. Use your hands, heart, brow chakra, or any other comfortable connection points.

10. Repeat this focus several times until you feel it is well established.

11. Attune once more and check either mentally or with dowsing techniques that the program is settled and has been activated.

12. Visually and mentally close, seal, heal, and protect the crystal structure that carries your program.

13. Repeat the whole process once or twice to reinforce your intent.

Healing with Crystal Pendulums

*P*endulum dowsing has a long history of use among healers of all types. As an assessment tool, learning to dowse is an essential skill for anyone wishing to work with crystals. It is well worth the time and practice in order to become confident and accurate in the use of pendulums. The skill needed for dowsing for information is largely one of mental attitude and correct procedure. There are also methods of using pendulums as tools for healing in their own right.

A pendulum is very simply a balanced weight on the end of a string or chain that allows movement. The actual swing or other movements of the pendulum are an amplification of minute physical or energetic changes within the muscles of the dowser. Like any other dowsing tool, the pendulum is an aid to recognizing changes in energy, so that they are shown in a clearly visible way.

Crystals interact dynamically with the human energy field, and when they are able to move through the aura, a powerful cleansing and balancing can occur. With the following techniques, the holder of the pendulum stays mentally neutral. No questioning is used or information sought. The pendulum is simply moved through the aura and left to swing in whichever way it wishes.

Any object moving through the auric field will have an effect of one sort or another. A crystal or gemstone is necessary to guarantee a beneficial healing effect. The most useful crystals to begin working with are clear quartz and amethyst. Both have a broad balancing effect on many systems.

BELOW *So long as it is a natural stone, healing pendulums can be of any shape or size to suit your needs.*

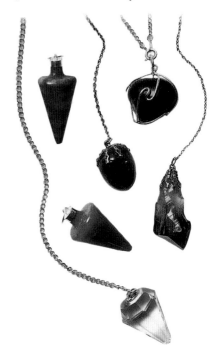

FIVE-LINE CLEARING METHOD

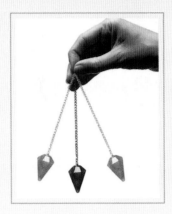

LEFT *Start off by guiding the pendulum into a neutral swing—a straight line to and fro.*

1 *Hold the pendulum lightly and firmly between your thumb and index finger. Keep your arm and shoulder relaxed and your body in a comfortable position. Your forearm should be held more or less level, with the wrist relaxed.*

2 *Before starting, consciously intend that the crystal pendulum will move away from the neutral swing only when it approaches an imbalance in the subtle bodies that can be corrected quickly and safely. This last point is important because it sets limits on a session that otherwise might last for a long time and release more stress than would be comfortable.*

3 *Start the pendulum swinging in a straight line, to and fro. This is known as the neutral swing. Any deviation from this simple swing will indicate that the pendulum is interacting with the energy fields in order to restore balance.*

4 *Move slowly in a line up the center of the body, beginning just below the feet, about 4 inches (10 cm) above the body. Whenever the pendulum swing moves away from neutral, just stay at that point until the swing returns to neutral. Occasionally, the pendulum will seem to slow and stop and then start to move in another direction. Make sure the pendulum has returned to a stable, neutral swing before moving on.*

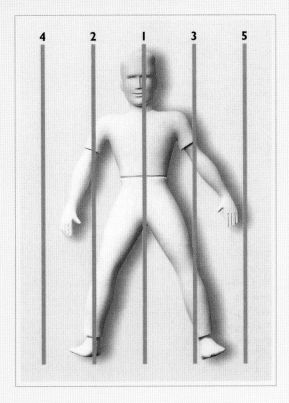

LEFT *Move on to swing the pendulum over a series of lines traveling up the body. It is useful to mark on a diagram of a body those places where the pendulum has picked up and corrected imbalances.*

5 When you have traveled up the whole body and reached a point approximately 12 inches (30 cm) above the head, start again at the feet, this time holding the pendulum to one side of the body. A line following the outside edge of the legs and torso is ideal.

7 For the last two sweeps, the pendulum is held farther away from the physical body but still parallel to the other lines. Here, it will be interacting mostly with the finest levels of energy within the auric field.

6 Repeat as before and then return to move up the other side of the body. The pendulum has now swept upward in three lines, covering all areas of the subtle bodies closest to the physical.

Variations

• The pendulum can be used to work even farther away from the physical body, creating profound clearing of the very fine subtle bodies that extend two further lines outward from the five lines and extend farther above and below the feet and head.

• Changing the height of the pendulum swing will interact with different energy layers. If there is a significant imbalance closer to the body, raising the pendulum up might help clear the subtle causes located in finer layers of energy.

• A pendulum made from a Herkimer diamond will detoxify energy fields effectively.

• Hold a lodestone stationary and move it slowly through the aura. Where it moves, there are electromagnetic imbalances, usually emanating from environmental sources. Or, alternatively, keep the lodestone swinging in a rapid circle and move through the aura. This will disperse any buildup of electromagnetic static around the body.

• Before starting the five-line clearing, think of the area or problem to be dealt with, such as the emotional body or the healing of an illness. The pendulum will then move only over relevant imbalances.

• Use the pendulum sweep to quickly assess which areas require work. Stone placements and other techniques can then be used to rebalance the body.

Massage Wands

*M*assage wands are a gentle and powerful way to introduce healing energies into the auric field. Wands are sometimes natural crystals that have had their bases smoothed and rounded, but most often they are cut from larger blocks of stone and are given a faceted point at one end and a rounded end at the other. This round end allows them to be used safely on the skin without scratching or irritating. The cool, smooth sensation they produce is extremely relaxing and they can be a useful adjunct to many forms of massage. Where there are areas of deep pain, lightly moving a massage wand over the area will help to relax and reduce the discomfort. Generally speaking, imbalances and tensions will be drawn out using small counterclockwise circles, but allow intuition and your body's own subtle senses to guide the movements of the wand.

ABOVE *Many crystal healers find that, as well as the natural crystals in their kit, shaped crystals serve useful purposes.*

Massage wands are also extremely effective tools for working within the subtle bodies. Their smooth, streamlined, highly polished shapes often seem to create less turbulence when moving through the aura than other shapes of stone.

Wand Method

The following method is an excellent way to become aware of your own intuitive skills while allowing profound healing on many levels. The deeper the healing work, the greater is the need for the healer to remain centered and grounded. It may be necessary to use a grounding stone or a grounding layout as a final procedure.

The principal purpose of this technique is to remove stress from the subtle bodies, at the same time aligning all energy fields. The wand is moved through the aura as is felt appropriate, but the following guidelines operate where personal intuition is absent:

1. Hold the wand comfortably, with the rounded end closest to the body, pointing outward.

2. Starting near the patient's feet and slowly moving up, make small, counter-clockwise circling movements with the wand 2 to 6 inches (5–15 cm) above the body.

3. The first part of this process is to slowly move up the body, unwinding any stresses and tensions. The speed at which you move or the order in which you proceed will be entirely up to you.

4. As you move the wand through the aura, you will experience a difference of quality in the movement of the wand or a sense of weight, lightness, stickiness, or even a difference within your own feelings. Wherever such changes are recognized, spend longer with the wand until it once again feels comfortable and smooth.

BELOW *The chiseled shape of a massage wand enters an aura with ease and lessens any disturbance caused by passing through it.*

5. Often the movement of your hand will want to change. Allow the movement that feels most comfortable to you. In this healing method, the only thing you can do wrong is to ignore your intuitive modifications.

6. When the top of the head is reached, change the position of the wand so that it is held with the point facing the body. The movement used should now be small, clockwise circles that recharge and energize the subtle bodies. Again variations may occur, although usually this second stage—moving from head back to feet—is a lot clearer and quicker to complete.

7. It is not very important in which hand the wand is held. Find the most comfortable position so that there is no physical strain in reaching over the whole auric field.

8. Make sure your patient is comfortable and ask them to let you know if they experience any strange sensations or if their mood or thoughts suddenly change. These will give further clues to the areas being released.

9. Be sure to make clear that any areas of imbalance identified will be on many different levels. One of the great strengths of crystal healing is that it can remove causes of potential illness long before it occurs on a physical level.

VARIATIONS

• Remember, working farther away from the body means that you will be interacting with the finest levels of awareness and thus potentially more powerfully. You can alter the height at which the wand is being held if you wish.

• This massage-wand technique can be used to great effect to speed up localized healing. Follow the same procedures as with whole body sweeps.

• Different crystal wands will work well on different levels. A variety of wands can supply a huge range of working possibilities.

• The size and length of the wand will affect the number of levels of energy it will work with at any one time, but always remember that a very large or heavy wand will be much more tiring to use and often much more fragile.

LEFT *Working on the top of the head. The use of massage wands can create deep states of altered awareness, so make sure the patient takes time to return to normal consciousness at the end of the session.*

MAKE SURE THE PATIENT IS COMFORTABLE

MOVE THE CRYSTAL IN SMALL, CLOCKWISE CIRCLES

TURN THE POINT TOWARD THE HEAD

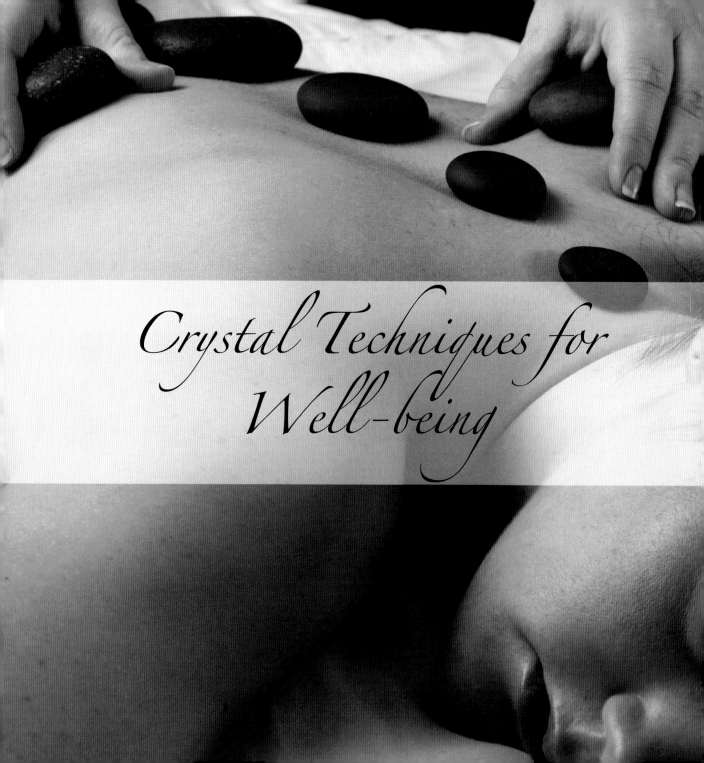

Crystal Techniques for Well-being

Emotional Stress

One of the greatest benefits of crystal healing is its ability to quickly and effectively reduce emotional stress. No matter what the level of an individual's health, emotional stress is a constant, energy-depleting drain of life force. Emotional stress includes the tiny, everyday nuisances and pressures as well as the large-scale events like illness, accidents, and bereavement. Each stress, unless released, adds pressure to existing weaknesses in the body.

Emotional stress burdens the body so that it becomes less able to repair itself or to repel invading microorganisms. Emotional imbalance floods the physical body with excessive levels of hormones, prevents proper absorption of nutrients, and creates tension and restricted circulation in muscle tissue. Existing stress at fine levels of awareness in the subtle bodies further prevents the dissipation of more surface stress. Emotional stress builds up chemical and energetic toxins.

Stress release using crystals doesn't require the conscious recall of an event. It can be likened to gently waking someone from a nightmare or a daydream. Before beginning any work to release stress, it is essential to make sure that it is an appropriate time to work on the chosen areas. Removing a lot of stress too rapidly can unbalance our lives to such an extent that it becomes very uncomfortable.

Emotional stresses tend to cluster together in pockets of associated events. The body may need to disengage itself from some of its older, less-raw emotional stresses before it feels comfortable addressing more current concerns.

Emotional Stress Release Technique

Sometimes it can be useful to precisely identify an area of stress that needs to be released. The following technique, based on kinesiology, can use either dowsing or muscle testing.

1. Find a strong indicator muscle *(see pages 135–137)*.

2. Lightly hold the slightly raised bulges on each side of the forehead between the eyebrows and the hairline. Retest the indicator muscle. If it is now weak, this shows that emotional stress is present and it is appropriate to release it.

3. The next step isolates the area of the emotions in which the stress is stored. Test each of the following words by saying them aloud and testing a strong indicator muscle. One or more words will weaken the muscle, indicating the areas of stress. The categories are: fear, anger, grief, joy, and sympathy.

4. Once the category has been found, next isolate the year in which stress is focused. Test by age, i.e. between 0 and 10, between 10 and 20, and so on, up to the person's present age. Sometimes other possibilities emerge, such as conception, birth, past, or future lives.

5. Find the focus of the stress: self, family, relationships, vacation, school, work, pets, and so on. In all of this testing, the stressful area will weaken a strong muscle. Write down all the information.

6. This information may help the person consciously remember the events, but it is not essential, as the stress will release automatically.

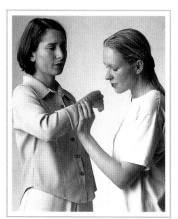

ABOVE *Begin by looking for a strong indicator muscle to enable you to identify the precise area of stress.*

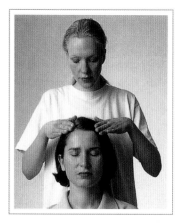

ABOVE *Holding the forehead points can create an energetic link where emotional stress can easily flow between healer and patient.*

7. Once the information is found, repeat all the factors aloud. This will remind the body of the exact stress to be released.

8. The patient sits or lies comfortably and thinks through or around the events.

9. While the person is thinking, the healer lightly holds the forehead with the fingertips of both hands. Alternatively, two crystals can be lightly taped in place.

10. The release can be carried out in silence, or the patient can report memories and sensations. In either case, the healer should regularly check how the patient is feeling. Make sure that both of you are comfortable before beginning, so the process is not interrupted.

11. There is usually a noticeable change of mood when the stress has cleared. A retest of the strong muscle, with the stress factors spoken aloud, should remain strong if the stress has been fully released.

12. Retest all five category words. You may now be able to release other stresses. If there is time to work further, repeat the procedure until all category words test strong.

13. Remember that this technique will allow you to work only with stresses that the body is ready to release at the time.

Procedures

Where a lot of stress has been let go, check again the overall balance of the chakras and, if necessary, clear any energetic debris out of the auric field using a massage wand or crystal pendulum. In this case, amethyst quartz will do or calming and gentle healing stones, such as carnelian, aventurine, jade, and smoky quartz. Drinking a little fresh water will help re-establish electrical balance and will also help flush out any released toxins.

Using a massage wand or crystal spheres can be another way to encourage this stress release. Work with the smooth surfaces of the crystal and lightly move over the skin of the forehead and face in small, counterclockwise circles, paying attention to the sensitive areas around the frontal eminences.

A sign of release of stress, tension, or a rebalancing of energies is a very long, deep breath, a sigh, or a yawn. Involuntary muscle twitching and unconscious movements of a hand or foot can often indicate release of stress. Occasionally, the twitch is clearly linked to the event that caused the stress in the first place. The clearest sign of stress release is a rapid fluttering of the closed eyelids. Crying and sobbing are also indicators of release and, should they occur spontaneously, try to make the person as comfortable as possible— usually by turning the patient onto one side.

Make sure there are plenty of grounding stones at the legs and feet to allow a rapid clearing of released energy and to help prevent the stresses from settling back into the subtle bodies.

TENSION RELEASE LAYOUT

1 *Place a rose quartz at the heart center and surround it with four clear quartz crystals with their points facing diagonally outward. This pattern will help release emotional blocks from the heart and disperse them so they won't settle elsewhere in the subtle bodies. The clear quartz crystal will naturally transform the disharmonious energy imbalances into a more life-sustaining quality.*

2 *At the second sacral chakra, below the navel, place a tiger's eye stone. Surround this with four clear quartz crystals with points facing diagonally inward. This part of the pattern helps give stability and grounding to the healing process. If the release is very strong, use extra grounding stones by the feet.*

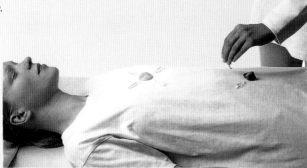

Layouts for Emotional Stress Release

*T*here are some layouts of crystals that can be very helpful both to release stress and to encourage positive change. With most crystal layouts described here, a short session repeated on a regular basis every few days conveys greater benefit than spending a longer time once in a while. In this way, the body becomes accustomed to the new balance of energy and is able to better maintain it during everyday activity. The longer the healing session, the more time it takes to integrate the new information, and therefore the benefits of healing take longer to emerge.

Personal Potential Layout

This layout helps clear emotional blocks so that suppressed or diverted skills can develop. The stones used are clear quartz and rose quartz to cleanse the auric field and re-establish self-confidence after emotional setbacks. If possible, this layout is best done lying on a yellow-colored cloth, which helps stimulate positive solar plexus energies and mental clarity.

The rose quartz stones are all placed in contact with the body. One is set at the top of the head, one is held in each hand, and one is placed on each foot between the tendons of the first and second toes.

The clear quartz stones are placed next to the body on each side of the head, level with the ears, beside the legs at knee level, and one beneath the feet. Crystals with points should face inward.

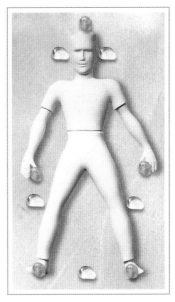

PERSONAL POTENTIAL LAYOUT

Five or ten minutes spent regularly in this energy pattern will help relieve stress.

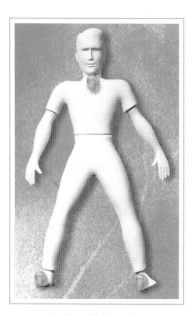

CONFIDENCE LAYOUT

Confidence Layout

The placement of stones here will help dissolve false inhibitions and stimulate motivation and drive.

Use a green cloth as a base color to focus the crystals' action on areas of balance, growth, and stress release around the heart chakra.

A rose quartz is placed at the base of the throat and one on each foot between the tendons of the first and second toes. Held in each hand is a clear quartz pointing away from the body. This both releases stress from the energy bodies and stimulates practical creativity and the desire to participate in the world.

Five minutes within these energies will help establish their beneficial effects.

Calming Layout

Moonstone helps calm the emotions and reduce stress. It relates both to the solar plexus, where it calms the digestive system and reduces fears, and to the sacral chakra, where it encourages the balance of all fluids within the body and helps dissolve emotional rigidity.

Using a blue cloth or background for this layout will emphasize the qualities of flow and peacefulness that the moonstones will direct into the subtle bodies.

Five moonstones of about the same size are used. If one stone is larger, place that at the top of the head, touching the scalp. On the front of the shoulders, in the hollow where arm meets torso, place a moonstone on each side. The remaining two stones are put on each hip bone. Some of these stones may need to be lightly taped in place.

This is a soothing healing pattern that induces a deep state of relaxation in which physical aches and pains can be relieved. Emotional worries tend to dissolve quickly from the mind. Occasionally, as the body releases stress and adjusts to the energies, there may be a sensation of pressure at the throat chakra. If it doesn't ease by itself, a light blue stone such as turquoise or blue lace agate will help the flow. It is easy to forget all sense of time in this energy net, so be aware that ten minutes will be ample to gain a healing benefit.

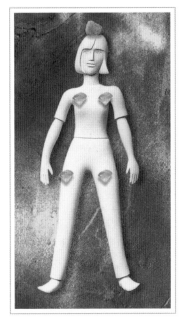

CALMING LAYOUT

Water Element Layout

The quality of water symbolizes the flow and flexibility that we require if we are to be healthy and grow in life. Water is linked with the emotions, and both water and the emotions share the tendency to move outward until they achieve a state of equilibrium. When this flow becomes blocked, pressure continues to accumulate, and, unless it is released, it can cause great destruction when it finally escapes.

Such emotional tension can lead to the sensation of being at bursting point, full of desperation and with feelings circling in on themselves. This layout of crystals may help release the internal pressure and establish a new state of balance.

Four rose quartz crystals are placed beside the feet and at the sides of the shoulders. This layout helps free the blocks from the energy systems of the body, particularly those to do with emotional conflicts.

A clear quartz crystal is laid at the thymus gland at the base of the throat. This helps strengthen the body's natural electromagnetic field and benefits both the immune and endocrine systems.

A sapphire crystal is placed above the top of the head to balance the subtle bodies, encouraging a healthy link between the physical, mental, and emotional systems. Specifically, this placement will ease depressive emotional states.

Using a blue cloth or surface on which the patient lies will help create a background energy of peacefulness, harmony, and communication.

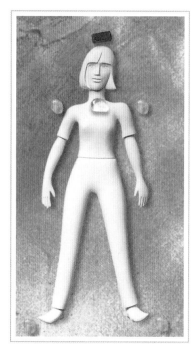

WATER ELEMENT LAYOUT

Meditation with Crystals

*M*editation covers a wide range of activities and states of awareness. It can generally be defined as a means of turning attention away from the conscious mind to focus on other processes. Meditation is often thought of as doing nothing. However, it would be more accurate to say that meditation is doing something different.

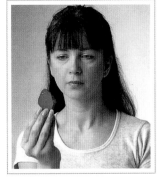

ABOVE *Gaze at the crystal for a few moments, then close your eyes and recreate the image. Open your eyes and repeat the process.*

Crystal, and quartz in particular, can be useful in many different types of meditations. The orderly energy structure of crystal naturally imparts a stillness and order to the subtle body system, and this in turn helps quieten the mind.

Problems are situations that have not been resolved by normal thought processes. By slightly altering our way of thinking—for example, by focusing the consciousness away from everyday issues—a solution can automatically arise.

Meditation Using Crystals

1. Place a crystal at a comfortable distance away from you, where your eyes can rest on it without strain. Begin by just gazing into the stone. Try not to blink. After a few minutes, close your eyes. In your mind's eye, try to recapture the image of the crystal. After a few minutes, open your eyes and gaze on the crystal again. You can repeat this procedure several times. Take some time before returning to everyday activity when you have finished.

2. You can adapt the gazing technique further by setting up certain parameters before you start the meditation. If you need help to solve a particular problem, you can think about that problem before opening your eyes to gaze

on the crystal. Before beginning, create a calm and comfortable atmosphere in which to meditate. Remain relaxed and let your thoughts flow. As the body relaxes and the mind calms, you may find a solution, or a solution may come to you later in the day.

3. This form of contemplation can also be used to find out more about how each crystal functions as a healing tool. Have several crystals on hand and explore them, one at a time, to reveal the individual healing properties of each one. This technique also helps you hone your own sensitivity to different crystals.

4. If you find it is particularly difficult to settle your mind, sit with a collection of stones and make patterns and shapes. You may find this active form of contemplation revealing as well as very relaxing. Try spreading your designs out to fill the floor and then sit at the center of the pattern for a few minutes.

5. Pick out two crystals that you feel are comfortable in your hands—for example, a clear quartz in one hand and a smoky quartz in the other. Begin with the smoky quartz in the right and clear quartz in the left. Sit for a few minutes and then swap the stones, putting the smoky in the left hand and the clear in your right hand. Note the differences. Try this with other crystals, noting and using the combinations that make you happy. Use one of them for a few minutes each day.

Guided Meditation

This meditation is based on one suggested by David Tansley, a British radionics practitioner and well-known researcher into subtle energies. It can be used as a refreshing, cleansing, and revitalizing exercise after a crystal-healing session or as a daily meditation. It can be very protective and centering and will encourage awareness of the whole self with its many different

BELOW *Sit with a different crystal in each hand while you contemplate for a few minutes, then swap them.*

CLEAR QUARTZ

SMOKY QUARTZ

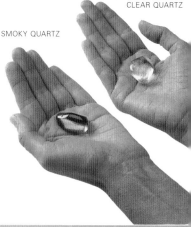

vibrational levels. Once learned, it can be worked through in a minute, quickly reminding us of our essential wholeness.

1. This meditation can be done seated or standing, whichever is more practical. Begin by finding a comfortable, relaxed position with eyes closed. Take a moment or two taking slow, deep breaths. You may hold a crystal of clear quartz if you wish.

2. Visualize in front of you three concentric, circular curtains of light flowing down and disappearing into the ground. The outer curtain, nearest to you, is a sparkling, golden yellow. The next curtain is a beautiful, soft rose- pink. The third and innermost curtain is a clear, electric blue. In the center of these three curtains of light, you can sense a bright source of radiant, white light, a sphere of energy suspended in the air.

3. Now see yourself in profile standing in front of the curtain of golden-yellow light.

4. Looking closely at the curtain, you can clearly see its downward movement, as if it were a waterfall of light.

5. In your mind, make the sound "Om," a traditional mantra, or word of power, that symbolizes the unity of creation.

6. Step through the curtain and, as you do so, visualize the light flowing completely through your physical and etheric bodies. See the solidity of your form melt into a body of golden light. Feel all the impurities and toxins lodged in the etheric body drop away from you onto the outside of the curtain where they dissolve.

7. Now find yourself standing before the curtain of rose-pink energies. This curtain represents your emotional body.

8. Once again, in your mind, sound "Om" and step forward into the pink energy. Feel it sweeping through your emotional body, like water cleansing

the fears, anxieties, and stresses. They all dissolve and drop away as you pass through the curtain.

9. Now you stand before the electric-blue curtain that is the mental body. Silently chant "Om" and step forward, letting all negative thought patterns and outmoded beliefs drop away behind you. Feel the weight of negative thoughts fall away.

10. In front of you now is the floating orb of radiant white light. This is the highest level of your own being, your true self, the core of your consciousness. Experience the clarity and wholeness flood through you, bringing with it understanding, peace, and love. Here at your center, stress and pain are unknown. Absorb the light into your newly cleansed aura and feel yourself expanding in a beautiful radiance of colors filled with vibrant energy and love. Nothing inharmonious or negative can approach you now.

11. When you are ready, bring your awareness back to the three curtains of light. Step through each one in turn. First blue, then pink, and last the yellow. Add an extra radiance to each as you pass through. You are now outside the curtains again.

12. Remember the light at the center of your being and allow yourself to expand to the whole of the universe, vibrating the "Om." As your energies return, become aware of your physical body. Take a deep breath, stretch, and, when you are ready, open your eyes slowly.

RIGHT *Your meditation will take you through various stages, dispersing negativity and strengthening energies.*

Goal Balancing

*G*oal balancing is one of the most useful methods available to the crystal healer. It can he used in a wide variety of circumstances and has the advantage of precisely focusing the healing processes in the desired direction.

Many complementary systems, among them crystal healing, work well when used as a preventative to reduce the likelihood of illness. Conventional medicine is structured to identify and treat symptoms of disease, and, as such, it has limited ability to work with wellness. Most doctors work from a state of disease, where the degree of disorder in the body has reached obvious levels.

With goal-balancing techniques, the crystal healer can work to reduce states of illness. More importantly, however, the healer can use them to help someone achieve any desired goal, whether it is a state of health, a lifestyle change, a long-cherished dream, or a state of mind.

Working with goal balancing is very rewarding because it helps remove blocks that are preventing someone from achieving their potential. Because the level of energy directed toward the goal is generally high, results become apparent quite quickly.

Goal Balancing by Chakras

1. Identify the goal as clearly as possible, once it has been established that a goal balance is appropriate. Sometimes the exact wording will be very important, and occasionally it may have peculiar grammar. What is important is that the stated goal is in a form the body recognizes and can work with. Be as

precise as possible. "Perfect health" is a wonderful goal, but for most people it will take considerable change to achieve. "Tolerance of noise" or "restful sleep" are goals that are more likely to show noticeable improvements over a short period.

2. Once the goal has been clarified, say it out loud to reinforce it.

3. Perform a simple, single stone chakra balance with the intention of balancing the chakras for the stated goal. Each stone chosen will then not only bring a general balance to the chakra but will also encourage those qualities in everyday life.

GOALS TO IDENTIFY

- Improve health conditions.
- Reduce fears.
- Improve creativity.
- Find or clarify spiritual direction.
- Improve emotional or mental states.

- Clear particular stresses.
- Become more effective at work.
- Build confidence for tests and examinations.
- Improve and understand relationships.

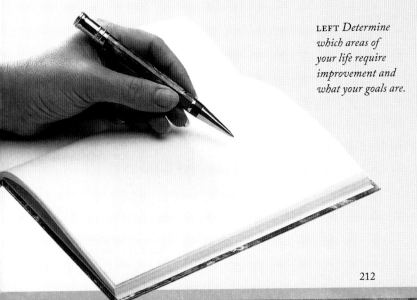

LEFT *Determine which areas of your life require improvement and what your goals are.*

ROBERT FROST TECHNIQUE

This is a goal-balancing technique based on a method devised by Robert Frost, a kinesiologist who has done extensive research into crystal energies. Muscle testing is ideal for this process because it clearly shows the patient how their body is recognizing the energy characteristics of each crystal. Dowsing can also be used if necessary. The premise is that every individual at a subtle energy level can recognize the most useful stone to help with any problem. This method simply lets the body choose that energy pattern.

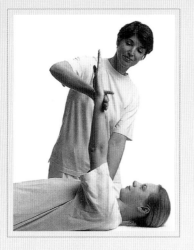

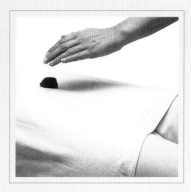

1 *After centering and grounding, check the patient for a strong indicator muscle and run through the initial balance to check for switching* (see pages 138–140).

2 *State the goal and check that it is appropriate for the present time.*

3 *Have a bag containing a good selection of different stones, one of each type.*

4 *Place the bag filled with stones on the navel area for a moment.*

5 Remove the bag and muscle test to see if one or more of the stones in the bag will balance the person for the stated goal.

6 If the response is negative, other stones will need to be found. If the response is positive, remove about half of the stones and put them to one side.

7 Place the bag with the remaining half of the stone selection on the navel and leave it there for a few moments.

8 Remove the bag and ask the same question. If the answer is "yes," then you know one or more of the stones now in the bag will assist in achieving the desired goal. If the answer is "no," you know that the selection you removed contains the required stone or stones.

9 Continue to divide the stones and retest until only one or two stones remain. These are the correct energies to help achieve the goal.

10 Finally, find out how they are to be used. If a stone should be worn, determine where on the body and for how long, day or night, and so on. If it should be kept elsewhere, find out the location. For example, should the stone be placed under a pillow, on a bedside table, or in the kitchen, car, handbag, etc.

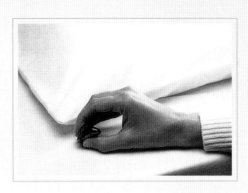

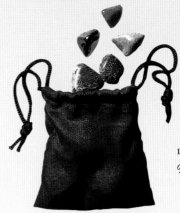

LEFT *A bag of stones.*

Absent Healing

Sometimes it can be advantageous to be able to work on healing someone who is not physically present. This is known as absent or distant healing. Absent healing can work very effectively, but it is not to be treated lightly and the normal safety measures should not be ignored. In fact, absent healing requires scrupulous adherence to the procedures of centering and grounding and careful use of assessment and balancing techniques. Failure to do this can lead to an absorption of emotions, or even disease patterns, from the absent person.

BELOW *To perform absent healing, you will need to collect personal mementoes (witnesses) of the patient.*

Thinking well of another person is the simplest absent healing of all. Gossip and other such negative character judgments not only depress the life force of the unwitting subjects, but also damage the speaker's energy structures as well. A blessing benediction and a careless curse can create endless ramifications of healing and disease. When asked by a student how to gain enlightenment quickly, one Master replied, "Just meditate regularly and never speak ill of others. Nothing else is required."

Asking permission of the subject may lessen the trap most healers will fall into at one time or another—the overwhelming need to bring about healing in order to lessen one's own pain at seeing the suffering of others. This self-absorbed state is wholly understandable but needs to be recognized and balanced with dignified restraint. Otherwise, it can easily lead to a false martyrdom, sacrificing one's own health and life for the sake of others people's.

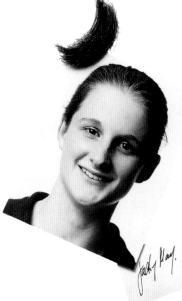

ABSENT HEALING PROCEDURE

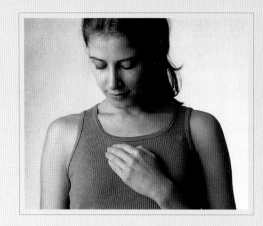

1 *Begin by centering and grounding yourself.
Tap yourself in. Check that your energies are
balanced and that you are ready, willing, and able
to do the proposed absent healing.*

2 *Check whether you need protection and support.
This is much more likely to be necessary in absent
healing work.*

FLAT-BASED QUARTZ   LOCK OF HAIR   MIRROR TILE

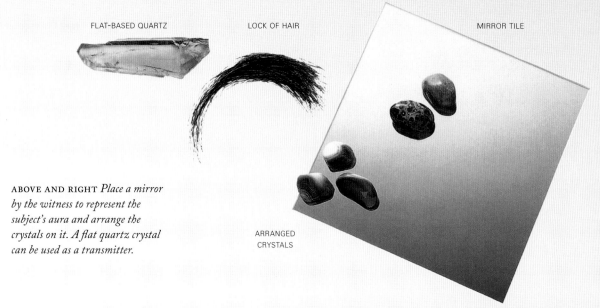

ARRANGED
CRYSTALS

ABOVE AND RIGHT *Place a mirror
by the witness to represent the
subject's aura and arrange the
crystals on it. A flat quartz crystal
can be used as a transmitter.*

216

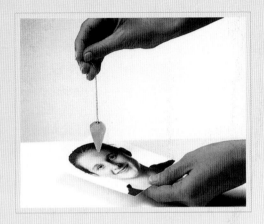

3 Hold the witness or touch it and allow time for your subtle perceptions to familiarize yourself with the energy pattern. One way is to put a pendulum into a circular swing. When it returns to a neutral swing, it indicates that the process is complete.

4 Use your skills to identify the best crystals to help heal and support the person. This step depends on whether any assessment is required or if healing energy is simply going to be given. At some stage, it will be necessary to determine what form the healing energy is going to take.

5 The crystals will then need to he placed on the witness and left somewhere undisturbed. Check to see how long the stones need to be in place. If several days or weeks are indicated, check again every day or so to see if any changes are needed.

How the crystals are arranged is up to your intuitive senses. A flat-based quartz crystal standing upright on or near the witness can act as an added transmitter. A small mirror tile or a slice of agate can represent the aura of the subject and stones can be arranged on it. When the process is complete, check your own energies once more. Use these methods to give yourself healing. A mirror or an outline sketch of a body with your name at the top will work. Place stones and work as if carrying out a normal crystal healing session.

The second requirement of absent healing is the use of a witness. A witness is some object or substance that carries the energy pattern of the person being healed. It allows an accurate assessment of what is required, and it functions like a homing beacon for the healing energies. A witness is usually a small lock of hair, a drop of blood, a photograph, or a signature. An accurate natal astrological chart is a unique representation of an individual's energy characteristics and can make an ideal witness.

ABSENT HEALING

The first rule of absent healing is to work only on someone who has given you permission to do so. This agreement ensures that the healer is not imposing in any way upon the free will of another and that the patient is fully aware and cooperating with the healing energy. In the case of those who are unable to ask for themselves, or with young children and animals, checking the appropriateness of any healing can be made through dowsing, intuition, or meditation.

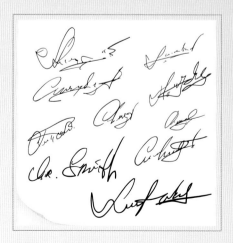

LEFT *For absent healing, you'll need something personal from the man or woman being healed. It can be anything from a lock of hair to a signature.*

Plants and Animals

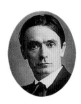

ABOVE *Rudolf Steiner made use of mineral and planetary influences.*

*P*lants have a natural affinity with the mineral kingdom. It has been suggested that understanding the astrological correspondences of plants, and linking them with appropriate gemstones, can strengthen their growth and yield. Crystals can also support your pets through times of illness, since animals respond very well to subtle forms of healing.

Plants

Plants introduce new minerals into the food chain. It is their root systems that break up the subsoil and rock by which minerals are transported to the topsoil. Vast quantities of minerals are added to fertilizers to improve crop yields. Unfortunately, this creates imbalances in ecosystems, which can lead to further impoverishment of the soil's fertility. A more subtle application of crystal and mineral energies can increase the health of plants without degrading the soil.

Rudolf Steiner, the founder of anthroposophical medicine, established a garden and farm regime that used organic and mineral substances, which were made effective through combinations of planetary and stellar influences together with positive intention and prayer. Linking plants with appropriate gemstones can improve their fertility. For example, plants ruled by the energies of the sun, such as corn and sunflower, would be energized by garnet and ruby. If these stones were placed near the plants, or if a gem remedy were used to water the soil, the mineral absorption would improve and the subtle life energy of the plant would also increase.

Experimentation in the field has indicated that certain rocks and crystal formations attract or amplify electromagnetic frequencies that encourage localized plant growth. The presence of a quartz crystal can amplify plant growth and adds a beneficial energizing effect. Emerald, and indeed beryl of any kind, is said to enhance all plants because it has a natural connection to the heart and the sun.

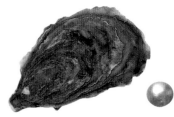

ABOVE *Oysters and pearls act as a conduit for the energies of other stones when they are pushed into the soil.*

Animals

Most owners are aware that pets are very sensitive to changes of atmosphere and can pick up frequencies far beyond the human range. This means they will sense the energy of crystals in an amplified manner as well. Caution is required when working in this way, however, so as not to disturb your pet unduly. Cats tend to be fussier than dogs, and most will be wary if a lot of crystals are placed near them. It will be very obvious if an unwell animal does

CRYSTAL FERTILIZERS

Pearl and oyster shells crushed and added to the soil are rich fertilizers and are also effective carriers for the energy of other stones placed in the soil for a specific purpose. Stones suggested are: pearl to be used with grains such as barley, millet, and rice; lapis lazuli and obsidian for desert plants and infertile soil; amethyst for wheat and oats; amber with trees whose sap is medicinal, such as birch, maple, and pine; jet to help shade-loving plants and mushrooms and to help prevent root disease; jade to help attune to the subtle realms of nature and as an overall amplifier of plant energy; turquoise to help plants recover from damage or disease.

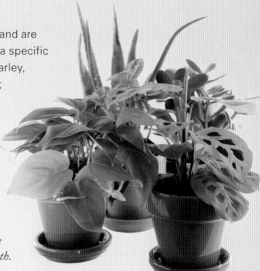

RIGHT *Slip quartz or beryl into plant pots and you will be rewarded by burgeoning growth.*

220

not appreciate this form of attention, but one that curls up and goes to sleep with crystals nearby has found that energy comfortable.

A massage wand or crystal pendulum can be an effective healing tool if your pet will allow you to use it. Work with it as you would on a person. Dogs and cats have chakras as well. Most four-legged animals have three main energy centers. They are at the top of the head, halfway along the backbone, and at the base of the tail. The whiskers, ears, and end of the tail are also areas that are especially sensitive to subtle frequencies.

If a particular crystal is needed by your pet, it can be placed safely in its bed or put into a small bag or pouch and securely attached to the collar. A tumbled stone can also be put in a silver spiral and suspended along with the name tag.

An effective method to give your pet a boost of healing energy is to use a gem water or gem essence. A few drops can be added to their drinking water, or you could place a couple of drops on your hands and stroke it through their fur or around their auric field, from head to tail, two or three times. If you are concerned about their health, it is wise to contact your veterinary practitioner.

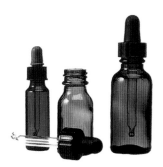

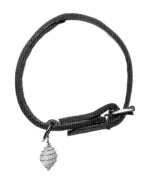

LEFT AND RIGHT *Pets can benefit from a securely placed crystal on their collar. Gem essences can easily be stroked through their fur or diluted in their drinking water.*

ANIMAL MAGIC

Animals are especially responsive to crystal healing treatment, probably because they have simpler, less convoluted mental barriers. Massage wands or pendulums work well, and particular crystals can be attached to their collars or placed in their beds.

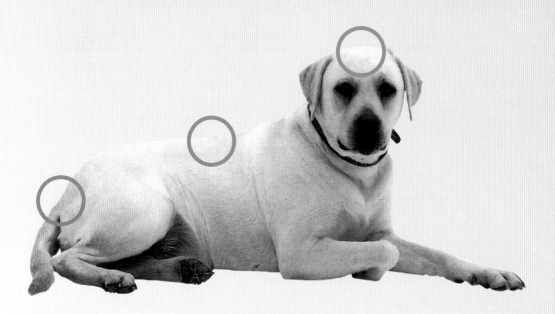

ABOVE *Animals have chakras: in dogs and cats, some of the main ones are on the head, middle of the back, and base of the tail.*

Carrying and Wearing Crystals

The earliest archeological evidence shows that mankind has always chosen to wear crystals, stones, and other magically precious items in order to absorb their beneficial properties. Today, wearing precious and semiprecious stones is widespread and popular. Wearing or carrying a crystal can be a helpful way to maintain the energy balance within the body.

Cleansing

Placing your jewelry on a cluster of crystals overnight will help remove any imbalances picked up during the day. This can be important when you have had a stressful day. Holding a stone under running water or cleansing it with incense or essential oil may also be necessary.

Some stones will be more prone to energy exhaustion than others. Generally speaking, the softer the mineral, the more quickly it absorbs energy patterns and the sooner it requires cleansing. Malachite, for example, is ideally suited to absorbing imbalances from painful areas of the body, but it will need recuperation after quite a short time.

The harder minerals like quartz, beryl, corundum, and diamond absorb energy to a lesser degree and will tend to cope for a longer time in stressed situations. However, when they do reach their limit, their natural broadcasting qualities will sometimes deflect disruptive vibrations into their immediate surroundings unchanged or even amplified. This is obviously not desirable.

Some minerals are effective at neutralizing strong, potentially damaging energy patterns, while not taking on the stress themselves. Crystals with parallel striations are useful in this respect. Tourmaline, topaz, rutilated quartz, tourmaline quartz, kyanite, kunzite, and particularly labradorite are excellent stones to wear in awkward, disruptive, or threatening situations.

Wearing Stones and Crystals

Stones will often change their appearance when they are worn. This can be a natural process, such as opal becoming more colorful as it warms up next to the skin or turquoise becoming greener by absorbing skin oils or perfumes. Quartz crystal that is cloudy may become clearer over time, perhaps as the minute water or gas inclusions escape through small fractures, or inclusions of liquid may expand or contract with changes of temperature. Some crystals have had their natural color enhanced by heat or dyes, and they can revert to

PROTECTIVE CRYSTALS

MALACHITE

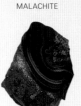

BLUE QUARTZ

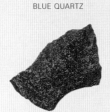

TOURMALINE QUARTZ

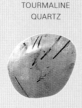

KUNZITE   TOPAZ

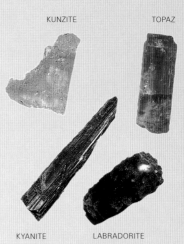

ABOVE *Malachite absorbs imbalances where you experience pain.*

ABOVE *Blue quartz also draws in energy, working over a longer period than malachite.*

ABOVE AND RIGHT *These stones are good for dispersing negative energy patterns. They help ward off threatening situations.*

KYANITE   LABRADORITE

their original appearance. Some crystals will fade when exposed to strong sunlight. Amethyst may do this, while others like kunzite may actually become more vivid. Sometimes, though, stones can change for no apparent physical reason. Very often in those cases, loss of color and an increase in fractures are a result of absorbing too much imbalance without the opportunity to restore equilibrium to the internal crystal structures. Such stones may never recover and are best given back to the Earth and buried.

Stones are often worn around the neck in the form of pendants. Depending on the length of cord or chain, different chakra points can be affected. Near the throat, a stone will modify communication skills and artistic expression. Placed close to the thymus gland, it will help the body's immune system and the meridians. Worn at the heart, the emotions will be affected, and, depending on the stone, vulnerability can be reduced. A stone worn around the solar plexus will interact with personal energy reserves, motivations, and power.

The upper chakras can be significantly affected by wearing earrings of crystal. For example, tourmaline or diamond can help alleviate structural tensions in the neck, jaw, ears, and skull bones.

Wearing gemstone rings can stimulate different meridian channels, depending upon which finger they are worn.

ABOVE *Wear one crystal at a time, or energies may interrupt each other.*

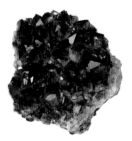

LEFT *The physical appearance of crystals can change over time. Amethysts, for example, can fade if they are exposed to strong sunlight.*

Carrying Gemstones

Where there is a need to carry a stone near a specific part of the body, a small bag or pouch can be attached to clothing using a safety pin.

At their best, crystals and gemstones can act as a support where the energy systems of the body need a little boost. However, they cannot replace long-term permanent change brought about through self-development and stress-release techniques.

Every stone you carry in your auric field modulates your energy. Wearing more than one or two stones at a time will often confuse the energy messages to the body, reducing the efficiency of the crystals and potentially disrupting their natural balance. Use crystal jewelry as a healing tool and treat it as you would gemstones in a crystal healing session—with care and precision.

Finally, don't wear or carry crystals all the time. There is a risk that you may become energetically or psychologically dependent on them. Every so often, have a couple of days where you do not use any crystal jewelry.

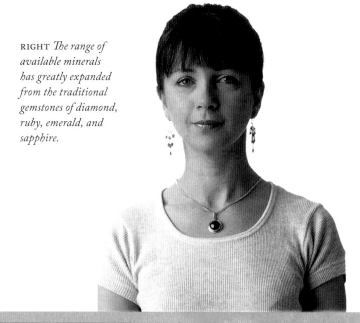

RIGHT *The range of available minerals has greatly expanded from the traditional gemstones of diamond, ruby, emerald, and sapphire.*

Crystals in the Home

The beauty of a cluster of crystals makes an effective decoration in all sorts of surroundings. The variety of colors and shapes offers a wide range of possibilities for creating an impressive highlight in any room. Careful placement of crystals around the home can also have a beneficial effect, since crystals alter the energy of a space dramatically, enlivening the atmosphere and neutralizing many negative effects.

Your home is an expression of your personality and how you like to be within yourself as well as how you would like others to see you. Adding an element of harmony and natural beauty automatically creates a positive psychological and emotional effect. A careful examination of those areas of your home that do not feel so comfortable will give a good indication of areas that need attention. The underlying energy and atmosphere of these areas can be improved by the placement of some crystals.

Once you have acquired basic dowsing skills, it is a relatively easy task to discern what areas in your home could do with the presence of crystals. There are no hard and fast rules as to where to place crystals. Use your own judgement. Clusters of crystals are impressive and have the ability to retain their own energy integrity much more easily than small single crystals. They will be able to transform more negative energy before they need to be cleansed again.

There are many reasons why crystals may be needed. At the simplest level, they can reflect light and brighten up shaded areas. Crystals hanging in a window can cast rainbows around the room as the sun shines in.

PRACTICAL APPLICATIONS

• Keep a bowl of tumbled stones or a favorite crystal by the telephone to prevent draining of energy from difficult phone calls. Holding the crystals will prevent overinvolvement or loss of perspective during the call.

• A crystal cluster near a computer screen or TV will help neutralize some of its electromagnetic fields. Cleanse the cluster regularly to reduce fatigue or irritability.

• A crystal can be the focus for a special place of meditation or remembrance. It will help cleanse and charge an atmosphere with life energy.

Before the advent of Austrian lead glass, all chandeliers were made from clear quartz cut into faceted drops that would beautifully reflect and augment the light from the candles.

Placement Exercise

Draw a floor plan of your home with all the larger pieces of furniture in place. Make a separate plan for each floor. You do not have to be absolutely accurate—approximate measurements are good enough.

With a pendulum or muscle-testing techniques, check each room to see whether it would benefit from crystals placed somewhere.

Mark the locations where the crystals need to be placed and then return to identify what sort of stone is needed and whether more than one would be advantageous, etc. Use color coding as your initial guide.

Cleanse all the stones you are going to use before placement, and every so often check them again to see if further cleansing is required.

This process will not necessarily remove or alter the nature of the energies in your home, but it will make them easier and less stressful.

BELOW *If the telephone is a potential source of stress, position calming crystals by it to neutralize disruptive influences.*

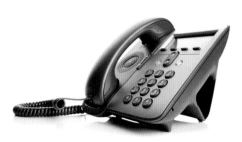

228

Crystals and Environmental Stress

*O*ne of the most significant factors affecting health today is the problem of environmental stress. The human body has adapted to its environmental conditions over millions of years. But the technological advances of the 20th century introduced a wide range of completely new factors to which the immune system has not had enough time to adjust.

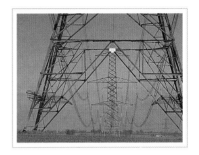

Everyday substances, such as plastics, electricity, radio, and microwaves, may have possible harmful effects. Petrochemicals, organophosphates, and radiation are demonstrably damaging to human tissue, yet they are now inescapable all over the world. These substances increase the stress loading on our systems, increasing susceptibility to disease.

ABOVE *Power lines are the source of vast electromagnetic fields, which are energy draining and detrimental to health.*

Electromagnetic Energy

The planet Earth has a natural electromagnetic energy called the geomagnetic field. All life has developed within this field and removal from it causes serious physiological problems. Man-made materials, such as metal girders, concrete, electric wiring, and plastic, can reduce this ambient Earth energy by shielding it or by setting up stronger electromagnetic resonances that may interfere with natural frequencies.

Every electrical device in the home creates a powerful electromagnetic field around itself. In someone who is run-down or especially susceptible, this can create a problem of entrainment. This is when the natural frequencies of the body become enmeshed with a stronger set of frequencies from an outside source.

There are some clear indications of susceptibility to electromagnetic stress, such as multiple allergic reactions made particularly worse in metal surroundings, sensitivity to thunderstorms, difficulties with fluorescent light, static electricity from clothes or car doors, intolerance to water, or a tendency to make electrical apparatuses break down or malfunction. A pendulum of magnetite or lodestone held steady will rotate in front of any part of the body under electromagnetic stress. Muscle testing will clearly indicate problem areas. Modern offices with computers, artificial lighting, tinted windows, air conditioning, nylon carpeting, and metal furniture can be disastrous for the energy system.

By amplifying personal energy fields, many crystals can help counteract the effects of environmental pollution. In very electrical environments, plastic buckets of salt water will help neutralize electrical resonance buildup, and clearing the aura with a pendulum of lodestone, magnetite, or copper every day will help restore natural frequencies. Move the pendulum in a circular motion and pass it through all of the auric fields several times.

Use the assessment procedure for protection and support or a goal balance to identify which crystals will be helpful.

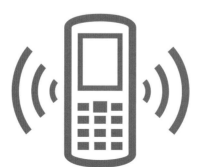

LEFT *The microwave radiations in cellular phones may disturb the body's chemical reactions.*

Crystals and Astrology

*T*oday, both Western and Eastern systems have merged to give gemstones for each month, planet, and zodiac sign. The reasons for attributing a stone to a particular sign can be various. Even a stone's color may link it to a planet. Copper minerals tend to be green, and the metal copper is said to be related to the planet Venus.

Each planet at the time of birth forms a unique relationship with all other planets, dependent not only on when but also on where you were born. The energies of the universe, represented by the 12 signs of the zodiac, are modified by any planet that happens to be between the Earth and the constellation at the time of birth, hence the Moon in Scorpio, the Sun in Leo, and the like.

The angles each planet makes in relation to others also alter personal energies in a natal chart. Some may amplify certain tendencies; others can create awkward juxtapositions of energy. The natal chart presents us with a toolbox of energies or a series of skills that we can develop or ignore.

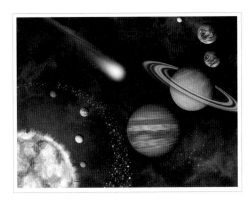

LEFT *Gemstones are closely associated with the planets in the solar system. Even a stone's color can link it to a planet.*

Healing with Astrological Layouts

The planets and signs continually circle around us, creating an everchanging pattern of cosmic energies, which sometimes create a sensitive time when they interact with our own natal chart details. Most of the time these transits pass by unnoticed, but occasionally they trigger periods of turbulence. If you suspect the influence of transits, carry or wear a piece of natural native copper. If this reduces the pressure you feel, it may indicate an active transit. Copper helps reduce the effects of difficult transits and amplifies positive astrological placements. Dowse a stone placement for the planets to help you to understand these energies. When dowsing, you need to have full astrological or astronomical information. A goal-balancing technique may also be helpful.

BIRTH ENERGY LAYOUT

One of the most powerful ways to experience your own natal chart energy is to create one large enough on which to place gemstones.

1 First, work out intuitively, or through dowsing or muscle testing, the most appropriate stones for each planet and sign.

2 Lay the 12 stones representing the zodiac constellations in a large circle on the floor.

3 Inside this circle, create a second circle with stones that represent the planets and place them in their appropriate signs according to your natal chart.

4 Dowse, intuit, or muscle test which is the most appropriate direction to lie inside the pattern.

5 Spend a short time inside the crystal energies a few times a month to familiarize yourself with this layout.

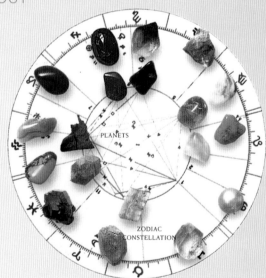

PLANETS

ZODIAC
CONSTELLATION

ASTROLOGICAL CORRESPONDENCES FOR PLANETS AND SIGNS

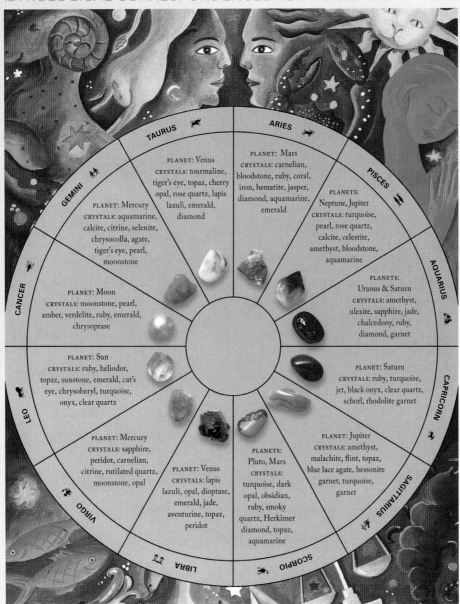

TAURUS

PLANET: Venus
CRYSTALS: tourmaline, tiger's eye, topaz, cherry opal, rose quartz, lapis lazuli, emerald, diamond

ARIES

PLANET: Mars
CRYSTALS: carnelian, bloodstone, ruby, coral, iron, hematite, jasper, diamond, aquamarine, emerald

GEMINI

PLANET: Mercury
CRYSTALS: aquamarine, calcite, citrine, selenite, chrysocolla, agate, tiger's eye, pearl, moonstone

PISCES

PLANETS: Neptune, Jupiter
CRYSTALS: turquoise, pearl, rose quartz, calcite, celestite, amethyst, bloodstone, aquamarine

CANCER

PLANET: Moon
CRYSTALS: moonstone, pearl, amber, verdelite, ruby, emerald, chrysoprase

AQUARIUS

PLANETS: Uranus & Saturn
CRYSTALS: amethyst, ulexite, sapphire, jade, chalcedony, ruby, diamond, garnet

LEO

PLANET: Sun
CRYSTALS: ruby, heliodor, topaz, sunstone, emerald, cat's eye, chrysoberyl, turquoise, onyx, clear quartz

CAPRICORN

PLANET: Saturn
CRYSTALS: ruby, turquoise, jet, black onyx, clear quartz, schorl, rhodolite garnet

VIRGO

PLANET: Mercury
CRYSTALS: sapphire, peridot, carnelian, citrine, rutilated quartz, moonstone, opal

SAGITTARIUS

PLANET: Jupiter
CRYSTALS: amethyst, malachite, flint, topaz, blue lace agate, hessonite garnet, turquoise, garnet

LIBRA

PLANET: Venus
CRYSTALS: lapis lazuli, opal, dioptase, emerald, jade, aventurine, topaz, peridot

SCORPIO

PLANETS: Pluto, Mars
CRYSTALS: turquoise, dark opal, obsidian, ruby, smoky quartz, Herkimer diamond, topaz, aquamarine

Divination with Crystals

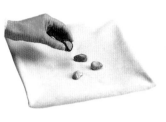

ABOVE *Stones can be cast onto a cloth, and a reading taken from the positions in which they fall.*

*T*hroughout the centuries, quartz crystal has been used as a way to reveal what is hidden either in the past, the present, or the future. Many tribal peoples specifically kept crystals for this purpose, feeling that the very nature of the stone allowed the mind to see beyond the physical into the realm of the spirits. Crystals can be used in two ways: scrying and divination.

Scrying, an Old English word meaning "to see or understand," is primarily a way to access the unconscious, or subconscious, mind. A crystal, or some other polished surface, is used to amplify or act as a screen for knowledge held in symbolic form within the mind. Scrying requires practice and discipline, but once the skill is acquired it can be used in many situations.

Divination uses the arrangement or pattern of objects and their interpretation according to pre-arranged guidelines or rules. The unconscious mind still plays an important part, but the process can be more objective. Divination with crystals usually takes the form of a certain number of different stones being randomly chosen or cast onto a cloth divided into sections. The information available to the crystal diviner depends upon the meaning that the stones and cloth have been given. The easiest way to attribute meanings is to use either the basic color of each stone as a guide or to use its healing qualities. For example, amethyst is violet and so is concerned with the imagination, fantasy, delusion, and achieving potential.

Simple Choosing Method

1. From a wide selection of different stones and crystals, ask a friend to choose four that attract her.

2. The first stone chosen represents her physical state. The second stone represents her emotions, the third is her mental state, and the last choice indicates her spiritual aspirations.

3. There is no need to tell your friend what each choice represents.

4. Decide beforehand that the selection will show what energies your friend needs in each area of her life, making it easier for you to interpret.

USING A CASTING CLOTH

Tossing or placing stones on a marked cloth can give a great deal of information about a situation. The design can be simple or very complicated. Areas where stones fall or are placed are important to the person at that time. Empty areas are not significant to the question.

CLOTH DESIGN
An area is divided into 12 segments based on the astrological houses. Each area represents an aspect of a person's life. Where the stones fall is interpreted in that light:

1. The self and personality
2. Possessions, feelings, beliefs
3. Associates, everyday communication, short journeys
4. Home, security, roots, mother or females
5. Creativity, leisure, risk-taking
6. Health, self-direction
7. Personal relationships and partnerships
8. Areas of change and transformation
9. Higher thought, learning, spiritual growth, long journeys
10. Career, outer persona, father figure or males
11. Social groups and friends
12. Hidden factors, behind-the-scenes activity

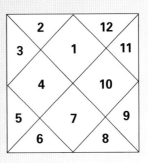

Scrying with Crystals

The objects that are used in scrying are various, but all have a quality of watery reflection and smoothness. Water, ink, oil, silver, mirrors, glass, gemstones, jet, obsidian, and clear quartz can all work effectively.

The mind should be in a state of awareness, a neutral receptiveness in which the mind is open and waiting to receive impressions in the form of sight, hearing, smell, or other sensory information. The conscious awareness takes a back seat and simply watches. Clear quartz will naturally take your mind to quieter levels of functioning where there is less surface chatter and a greater coherence of the brain waves.

Where quartz will quieten and balance the mind, allowing an expansion of awareness, a surface such as polished obsidian will work in the opposite way. Obsidian has no crystalline structure. It is amorphous. Gazing into an obsidian crystal can be compared to the effects of white noise where all sound frequencies exist but none predominates, leaving the mind unable to focus on any one sound. The best scrying tool is one with no internal forms. A small clear sphere can often be more effective than a large one filled with interesting patterns. Obsidian spheres, cabochons, or disks are usually less expensive than those of quartz.

Procedure

1. Center and ground your energies.

2. Spend a few minutes performing some sort of quiet meditation.

3. Place the crystal in a position in which you will see no reflections. If you are using an opaque reflective surface, look through the surface as if you were staring into the depths of a dark pool.

4. You might prefer to work at night or in a darkened room.

5. A black or dark blue cloth can be put around the crystal to reduce reflection and glare.

6. Take a minute or two to formulate your question clearly in your mind.

7. Focus the gaze into the center of the crystal or through it.

8. If you see clouds or mist of different colors continue to look through the crystal.

9. With practice, images will appear and sometimes sounds or smells may be noticed. Register these sensations without losing focus.

10. Remember that what appears is your unconscious mind's response to the particular question. The more precise the question, the easier it will be for you to interpret the images.

11. If you begin by focusing on a particular time or place, it will be easier to remain neutral.

12. When the time is up, remember to ground and center yourself.

RIGHT *Block out intrusive distracting light by using a dark cloth or by working in a darkened room.*

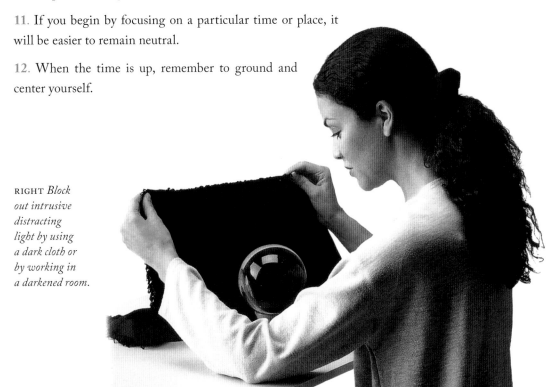

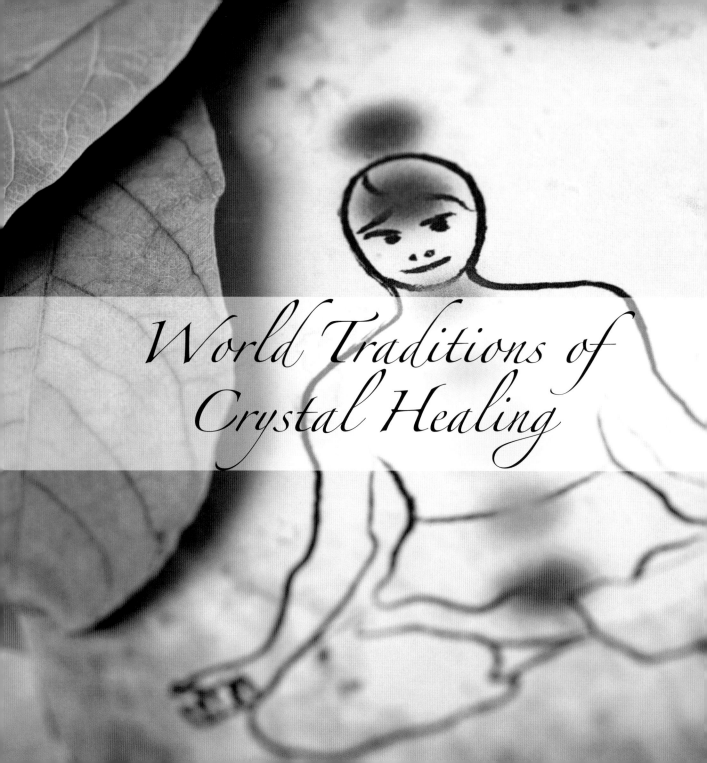

World Traditions of
Crystal Healing

The Stone Millennia

*I*f the whole of human history were scaled down to a year, only in the beginning of July would the simplest stone tools be found. As the year progresses, these tools become refined and specialized until finally, on the last day of the year, late in the afternoon, agriculture would begin and shortly after that, the Bronze Age. That evening, the Iron Age and Christianity would emerge, and only as the year came to a close would the Industrial Revolution burst forth. The 20th century begins just before the stroke of midnight. Such a view of time really puts the human relationship with stone into a proper perspective.

For these many thousands of years, humanity has familiarized itself with the uses and properties of stone. Tools were made from flint throughout the Stone Age. Great skill is evident in the making and shaping of these pieces. The Solutrean culture of south-

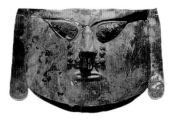

LEFT Stones and metals were fashioned into ceremonial art and decorative objects. This Peruvian burial mask was placed on rulers and chiefs and has copper inlaid eyes.

western France, about 20,000 years ago, produced exquisitely made laurel-leaf blades that may have performed a special ritual function.

In the Neolithic period, stone is associated with ritual burials. Jade was especially valued for making ceremonial axes polished to a mirror finish. Obsidian has also been found in Neolithic sites made into razor-sharp blades and mirrors. These materials continued to be sacred for many thousands of years. Jade became the most highly regarded stone of Imperial China, as well as South America and the islands of the Pacific. Amber has been found associated with burial sites of the megalithic and Neolithic periods. Easily worked, translucent, and richly colored, amber is found around the Baltic Sea, which became the focus for trade routes that covered the whole of Europe.

Perhaps the most sacred stone of all, with a history that goes back 100,000 years, is red ocher, the earthy iron ore often associated with hematite and magnetite. From Africa to France to Wales, red ocher has been found in the graves of Neanderthal peoples, and later, in the burials of Cro-Magnon man, or modern Homo sapiens. Red ocher is a substance associated with life energy, power, and the sacred.

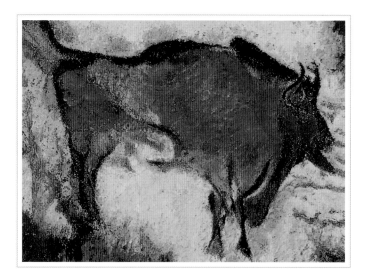

LEFT *The earliest cave art was painted with sticks dipped in colors made from ground-up minerals.*

Australia and Southeast Asia

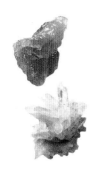

*T*hroughout this region, crystals are an essential part of the initiation rites of healers and shamans. The Australian Aborigines see crystals as sacred, associated with the Rainbow Serpent, an important mythological figure. On the Malay Peninsula, healers use quartz crystals to locate sickness in the patient and to find out how it can be removed. In Borneo, the shaman has "light stones" that are able to show whatever is going on in the patient's soul and can lead the shaman to where the lost soul is trapped.

ABOVE *Malaysian shamans believe that spirits in the air cut quartz crystals out of the sky for them to use in healing ceremonies.*

For the Australian Aborigines, the supreme god Baiame is the source of many healers' and magicians' power and is connected with quartz crystal. Baiame's throne is made of clear crystal, fragments of which are said to have fallen to Earth, where they can still sometimes be found. Here are the associations with rainbows, water, rain, clouds, and heaven, which link to quartz crystals as belonging to the upper world of the spirits and ancestors. They are considered solidified light.

In order to become a shaman, it is necessary to be filled with the solidified light of quartz crystal. This process fills the shaman with the substance of the sky, enabling him to journey whenever there is need. The Wiradjuri shamans put rock crystals into their apprentices' bodies and make them drink water in which crystals have been placed. This is said to enable the apprentice to see spirits. When he is ready to be taken by the shaman to Baiame, the Supreme Being, he is given some crystals and shown how to use them. He is then returned to his campsite and left in the top of a tree. These initiations largely take place in spirit journeys, but the abilities and healing skills learned there can be of real value to the tribe in everyday reality.

On the Malay Peninsula, the healer also uses quartz crystals that have been cut from the sky and given to him by the spirits of the air. The shaman might also make them from magically solidified water. Because they come from the sky, the crystals are able to show the healer and shaman things that are happening here on Earth. For example, where the sickness is in the patient and how it can be removed.

In Borneo, the shaman's "light stones," or crystals, are used in healing rituals that are carried out at night. First, crystals are rubbed over the patient's body and then, while onlookers chant rhythmically, the shaman dances until he falls exhausted and his spirit flies off to retrieve the patient's lost soul.

The Aranda of central Australia say that the candidate is taken by spirits into their caves, where all his internal organs are removed and replaced by "atmongara," or fragments of quartz.

A medicine man can also be created by other experienced elders. Taken to a solitary place, old men rub the candidate's body with rock crystals, press quartz into his scalp, pierce a hole under one fingernail, and make an incision in his tongue. He is decorated with symbols representing the spirits of Dreamtime, surrounded by lines that symbolize the magical crystals now in his body.

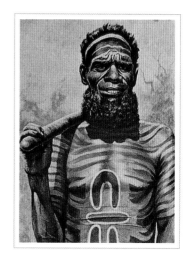

RIGHT *To become a shaman, the candidate undergoes a ritual where quartz crystals are used to prepare him for office. Magic crystals are absorbed into his body. This Aboriginal shaman displays extensive body painting.*

The Americas

*A*mong the native tribes of North America, crystals are held in high regard as objects of great healing and spiritual power. They are considered different from other stones and were known to some as *wii-ipay*, or "living rocks." Native burials as old as 8,000 years have been found to contain quartz crystals.

Present-day Yuman or Paipai shamans keep quartz crystals with them in deerskin pouches. As a protector and guardian, the stone's advice is sought continually in order to understand and work with the world of the spirits. Rattles used in dance and healing ceremonies to summon helpful spirits are often filled with small, round pebbles of quartz.

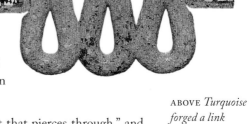

ABOVE *Turquoise forged a link between the earthly and the spiritual and was used on religious artifacts.*

The Cherokee name for crystal means "light that pierces through," and quartz was seen as a primary tool for revealing information and conveying messages. Sometimes the crystals would be positioned so that they caught the sun's first rays. Where the light from the stone fell indicated the required answer. Healers would warm a crystal over a fire and then lay it over a patient's body, looking through the quartz to determine the main areas of illness. Crystals were also rubbed between the healer's hands and then placed on a patient's body to remove pain.

The coastal Miwok near San Francisco had a very large quartz crystal of great power. On special occasions, it was "woken up" by a shaman, who would go to a particular rock and strike the crystal as hard against it as possible. Tribal tradition was that if the crystal shattered, the world would end.

Turquoise was a stone held in the highest regard by Central American Indians. It was used exclusively for decorating the images of their gods and for offerings. The tribes of the Southwest United States also value turquoise for its protective and strengthening qualities. Turquoise is seen as a link between heaven and Earth. The Apaches considered turquoise an essential part of the shaman's equipment, and hunters also wore the stone to protect themselves and to improve their chances of success.

Of special significance to all the tribes of North America is a quarry in Minnesota where, for centuries, people have dug out pipestone—a rich, red, soft stone also known as catlinite, from which the bowls of their sacred pipes were carved. Pipestone is considered to be the blood of the Earth and the people. The bowl represents the Earth, and the stem symbolizes the heavens. Quartz, turquoise, and pipestone have enabled generations of tribespeople to maintain their strong links with the spirits and their ancestors.

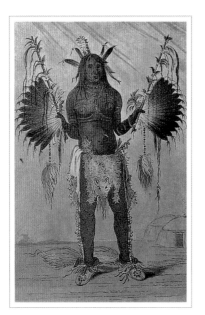

LEFT *Shamans used crystals for diagnosing and curing illness, as well as to find answers to questions.*

Central and South America

*I*t is clear from what remains of the impressive and mysterious cultures of Central and South America that stone-working was a valued craft. Many turquoise, obsidian, and jade objects have been found, as well as a few gold artifacts that escaped being shipped to Europe to be melted down.

Mica played an important role in the ritual procedures of the builders of the ancient city of Teotihuacán in Central America. The large central Pyramid of the Sun was originally capped with mica that would have reflected sunlight like sheets of glass. The nearby Mica Temple contains two hidden, massive slabs of mica, which were mined in Brazil, 2,000 miles away. Mica must have served more than a decorative function.

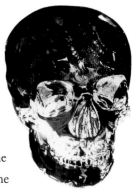

ABOVE *A crystal skull discovered in Central America. Crystals reflect light, mirroring the need to live in harmony with the energies of the universe.*

Jade is also found to be associated with religious and royal sites. At the Mayan city of Palenque in Mexico, there is a famous building known as the Temple of Inscriptions. Here, the Sun Lord Pacal was buried in 683 C.E. Two carved jade figures were found at the entrance to his tomb. The king was found wearing jade ornaments, including jade rings on his fingers and a necklace of jade beads around his neck. He wore earrings made from mother-of-pearl and held a piece of jade in each hand as well as one in his mouth. His face was covered with a death mask decorated with a mosaic of jade, obsidian, and white shell.

Quartz beads are often found in Central American burials, but rarely have large finds been made. However, a Mixtec grave found at Monté Alban in Central America was filled with many gold ornaments, pottery, and precious stones. The body had been buried wearing crystal beads, crystal earrings, and a crystal lip plug, all the insignia of the highly regarded astronomer caste. The most unusual find was a unique carved goblet or drinking vessel of clear quartz.

Farther south, among the tribespeople of the Colombian rainforests, quartz crystal is regarded as condensed solar energy in which a shaman can detect many different colors or energies that can be manipulated and balanced in order to ensure continuing harmony and abundance within the environment.

Shaman priests have learned how to use power stones and work in harmony with them. They are kept carefully wrapped in special cloths. These healing stones may look no different than garden or beach pebbles, but for the healer who has meditated and worked with them for many years, they are imbued with universal energy that can be called on to both locate, and remove, illness.

RIGHT *The Kogi of Colombia consider quartz and emerald to have religious significance, affecting fertility, healing, and order.*

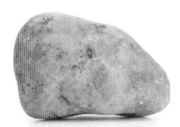
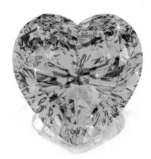

Use of Gemstones in Tantra and Ayurveda

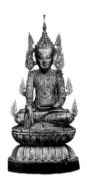

ABOVE *The ultimate goal of healing in these traditions is the end of all suffering—complete realization and enlightenment.*

The use of gemstones for healing has the longest-recorded history in India and may have influenced European systems via Greek and Arab trade contacts. The origin of gemstones is described in many ancient texts. In one text, the light that spreads out from the Creator of the Universe is reflected and transmitted to Earth through each of the planets. These rays are collected by gemstones and radiated into their surroundings to energize anyone nearby. In another text, gems were said to be created from light emanated by the planets, each having one of the colors of the rainbow.

Other descriptions in ancient Indian texts include an account of a supernatural being who offers himself for sacrifice in order to save the balance of creation, and whose remains are then converted into the "nine gems of eighty-four types." His blood becomes rubies, his teeth pearls, his eyes blue sapphires, and so on. As a logical progression from this image, gemstones were seen as being able to help specific parts and tissues of the body.

Gem powders and oxides are used to make sacred images and ritual patterns that contain beneficial energies. Crystals and gemstones are also used to make religious statues, prayer beads, and amulets because they are more powerful than most other materials, such as metal, and confer greater benefit.

Talismans are still made according to strict principles. In order to retain the maximum benefit, the appropriate crystal is selected and bought when the most favorable planets and constellations are at their greatest influence. The stones, which should be perfect in color, flawless, and of a correct weight, are set in metals of specific shapes. The metals or stones are inscribed with sacred designs, and the talisman has the prescribed number of repetitions of mantra recited over it. The use of talismans developed from ancient practices where deities and planetary energies were invoked using patterns of gemstones to create complex colored thangkas and mandalas. These devices were used to act as a focus for both contemplation and meditation.

AYURVEDIC GEMS OF THE NINE PLANETS

There are many ways to determine which gemstone will be the most beneficial. The stone representing the sign in which the Moon is placed is often used. The Moon represents the psyche and the underlying drive of a person. Some astrologers, however, prefer to check whether the Moon is in a supporting position in the first place and, if it weakness, will suggest a stone that will support the Moon's energy. Wearing a gemstone increases the energy of its related planet, so if the planet is not in a good position, the situation can be made worse. An experienced astrologer will select the most suitable stone after analyzing the natal chart.

PLANET	GEM	SUBSTITUTE GEM
Sun	Ruby (manikya)	Garnet, star ruby, red spinel, red zircon, red tourmaline, rose quartz
Moon	Pearl (mukta)	Moonstone, quartz
Mars	Coral (prawal)	Carnelian, red jasper

Early writings state that gemstones absorb and transmit the energy of the planets and are able to absorb negative energy, transforming it for use in the body. Astrologers and healers elaborated this system so that they could compensate for the deleterious effects of the planets' positions in someone's natal chart. A skillful astrologer will consider all planetary placements as well as favorable constellations and will balance this with the needs of the client. The most beneficial stone will be selected after careful scrutiny of the natal chart and patient requirements.

PLANET	GEM	SUBSTITUTE GEM
Mercury	Emerald (markat)	Aquamarine, peridot, green zircon, green agate, jade, green tourmaline
Jupiter	Yellow sapphire (pushpraga)	Yellow pearl, yellow zircon, yellow tourmaline, topaz, citrine
Venus	Diamond (vajra)	White sapphire, white zircon, white tourmaline
Saturn	Blue sapphire (neelmani)	Blue zircon, amethyst, blue tourmaline, lapis lazuli, blue spinel
Rahu*	Hessonite (gomed) [zircon]	Hessonite garnet
Ketu*	Cat's eye (vaidurya) [chrysoberyl]	Tiger's eye

*Rahu and ketu are lunar nodes associated with eclipses.

There are many traditional prohibitions regarding the wearing of gemstones, and rarely are stones able to be worn together. However, there is one arrangement that includes all nine planetary gemstones made into a ring or necklace. Based on a traditional design, it balances all influences together into a harmonious whole. The nine gems, the navratnas, are those with planetary influences. The remaining 75 other traditional ratnas or gems are mostly semiprecious stones used in medicine and healing.

In Ayurveda, these semiprecious stones are associated with the three energies of the body, the three doshas, which are pitta, vata, and kapha, representing the qualities of heat, air, and water. Health is maintained while the doshas are in balance; illness comes about through an imbalance in one or more doshas. Gemstones can be used to balance the doshas. Gemstones are powdered, mixed with honey or cream, and given by mouth. Gem waters are also used. A copper or silver vessel is filled with water, and the appropriate gemstone is placed in it overnight. In the morning, it is divided into three doses to be taken during the day.

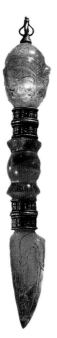

LEFT *A* phur-bu, *a silver and rock crystal ritual dagger used by Tibetan lamas to demarcate protective boundaries.*

The Biblical Tradition

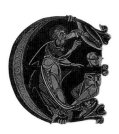

*T*he Bible contains references to crystals and gemstones in many places. Sometimes the writer uses familiar stones as an effective way to describe color. In other places, gemstones are used to suggest great riches and wealth. There are specific instructions for religious vestments and the stones they should contain. Finally, there are descriptions of visionary experiences of heaven and the spiritual realms.

In Exodus, Chapter 28, the Lord gives very detailed instructions on how to make "the breastplate of judgment" for the High Priest:

"And thou shalt make the breastplate of judgment with cunning work... and thou shalt set it in setting of stones, even four rows of stones: the first row shall be of sardonyx, a topaz, and a carbuncle... And a second row shall be an emerald, a sapphire, and a diamond. And a third row a ligure, an agate, and an amethyst. And a fourth row a beryl, and an onyx, and a jasper: they shall be set in gold in their enclosings."

In the Book of Job, precious gemstones are used to emphasize both the richness of the Earth and the order placed upon it by the Creator, and as a metaphor for material riches: "For the price of wisdom is above rubies. The topaz of Ethiopia shall not equal it, neither shall it be valued with pure gold."

The visions of Ezekiel and of John, in Revelation, use crystals and gemstones to communicate the richness and opulence of the experience. Ezekiel's vision of the heavenly beings is awesome: "And I looked and, behold, a whirlwind came out of the north... and a fire infolding itself... as the color of amber... And the likeness of the firmament upon the heads of the living creature was ... the color of the terrible crystal..."

The striking visions of John the Divine, as described in the Book of Revelation, were represented extensively in art throughout the Middle Ages in Europe. John's description of a new heaven and a new Earth, couched in the language of crystals, legitimized the lavish use of precious gems and metals in the Church. This allowed a burgeoning of creativity within the whole spectrum of religious life:

"And one of the seven angels... showed me that great city... And the foundations of the wall of the city were garnished with... precious stones. The first foundation was jasper; the second, sapphire; the third, a chalcedony; the fourth, an emerald; the fifth, sardonyx; the sixth, sardius; the seventh, chrysolite; the eighth, beryl; the ninth, a topaz; the tenth, a chrysoprase; the eleventh, a jacinth; the twelfth, an amethyst."

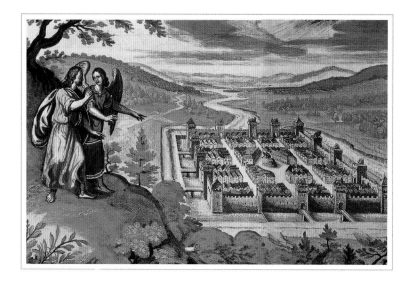

LEFT *In the Book of Revelation, John had a vision of a new heaven and a new Earth, containing a sumptuous array of crystals.*

THE ATLANTIS TRADITION

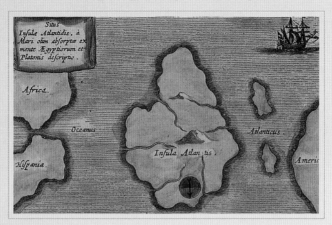

RIGHT *In the legendary civilization of Atlantis, crystals were used to generate energy and for healing.*

The legend of Atlantis and other civilizations of the distant past carry little credence in academic circles, although increasing research suggests the date for antiquities such as the Sphinx in Egypt is far older than most historians believe. For the present, Atlantis remains a powerful myth. Whether described as an island in the Atlantic or a planet now destroyed, the stories are often similar. There are descriptions of huge crystals, initially used for communication between dimensions, that were developed to generate power and energy throughout Atlantis. The Firestone, or Great Crystals, were housed in a dome that could concentrate the sun's rays into the crystals, creating tremendous energy. Some sources describe development of the use of crystals from an earlier civilization called Lemuria. Here, the inhabitants dwelled close to nature and experienced multidimensional consciousness, where awareness of both physical and subtle dimensions existed simultaneously. Gemstones were used to focus and modify consciousness, assisting the physical energies of the body. Atlantis developed from a Lemurian colony and tended toward a higher, technologically structured society. The harmony with the natural surroundings became disturbed, causing new health problems. Gemstones were used in specialized healing techniques, as well as in the modification of the genetic codes of humanity. There are descriptions of special healing chambers with walls made of quartz crystal in which people could enter to receive healing from large wandlike crystals or alternately go deep into meditation and experience higher forms of consciousness.

RIGHT *The Atlantis crystal groves were said to contain myriad crystal arrangements, including rubies, emeralds, amber, and lapis lazuli.*

RUBY

LAPIS LAZULI

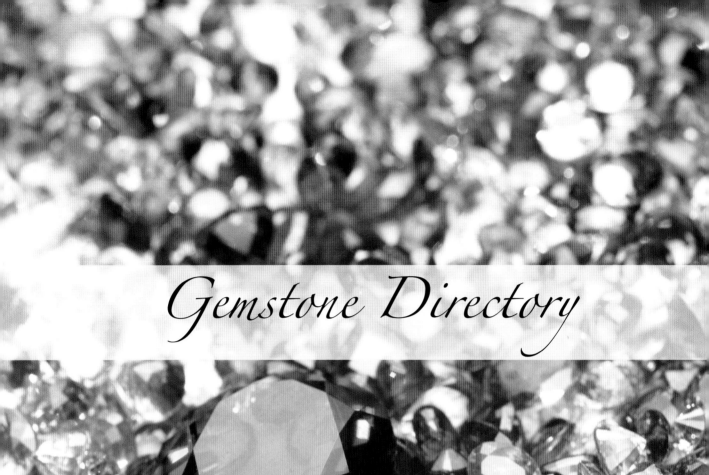

Gemstone Directory

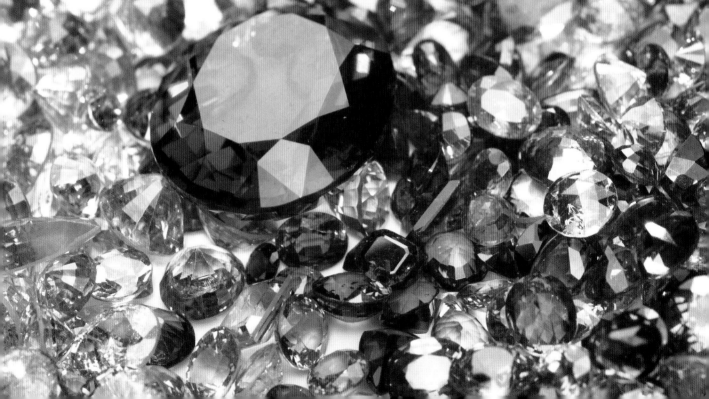

This directory is to help you identify some of the most useful crystals and minerals used in crystal healing. Because so much depends on the interaction between the energy of the mineral and the makeup of the individual, it is unwise to attribute specific healing properties to a stone. General tendencies are given here that, together with information that can be surmised from other characteristics such as the crystal system and color, can help the crystal worker ascertain what might be happening at energetic levels during a healing session. This directory is by no means an inclusive survey; there are thousands of minerals known, and several dozen new ones identified each year. Although every mineral has a potential for influencing health and well-being, the delicacy, rarity, or toxicity of some makes them impractical for general healing.

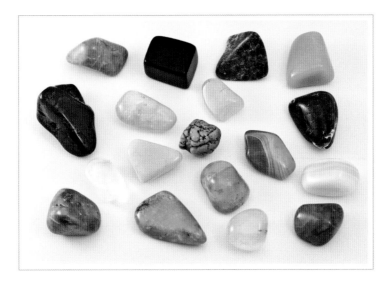

LEFT
A collection of polished gemstones.

LUSTER

Luster describes the way in which light is reflected away from a gemstone. The following examples are taken from the main categories of luster:

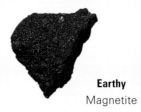

Earthy
Magnetite

Greasy
Blue calcite

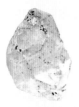

Adamantine
Diamond

Silky
Tiger's eye

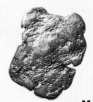

Metallic
Copper

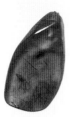

Resinous
Amber

Vitreous
Tourmaline quartz

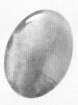

Pearl
Opal

Qualities and Attributes

Each crystal system tends to modify energy in particular ways, so the external shape that reflects the internal structure of a crystal will give some indication of its qualities as a healing tool.

Chemical Formula

The chemical formula of a mineral shows the complete makeup and relationship of elements within a crystal or rock. From this formula, it is easy to see how simple or complex a mineral may be. The formula also identifies similarities between different minerals and, in a few cases, where different minerals have exactly the same constituents arranged in different patterns.

Hardness

The hardness of a mineral shows first how delicate it may be. Softer stones will get easily damaged by careless handling. However, even hard minerals may be brittle and fracture easily. Soft stones tend to be better at absorbing energy than hard stones, which are effective amplifiers and broadcasters of energy.

Hardness is measured by the Mohs scale *(see box on pages 258–259)*, which was devised to aid identification of minerals. It indicates degree of hardness by a higher number. A sample with a high number will scratch all stones of a lower number.

RIGHT *Diamonds are the hardest natural substance.*

Luster

Luster *(see box on page 256)* is the way light reflects from the surface of a gemstone. The most frequently used descriptions are:

• **Adamantine:** Like a diamond, very hard and brilliant.

• **Vitreous:** Like glass, shiny but without brilliance.

• **Pearl:** Like pearls—a soft light, perhaps with iridescence.

• **Silky:** An uneven, rippling play of light, caused by irregular crystal structures beneath the surface.

• **Greasy:** Feeling moist, slippery, or slimy to the touch, may look wet.

• **Resinous:** A dull, sticky-looking surface, like amber or violin resin.

• **Earthy:** Dull and nonreflective.

• **Metallic:** Shiny and reflective.

Color

The colors listed under each mineral in this directory are those commonly seen. The actual color of a mineral is determined by a scratch test, where a sample is drawn across a plain unglazed porcelain tile. The color of the dust left behind is the true color of the mineral.

ABOVE *To identify a crystal's true color, scratch it across a plain, porcelain tile and examine the color of the remaining dust.*

Chakra and Subtle Body

Where there is a clear relationship between a stone and a chakra or subtle body, it is indicated in the directory. This in no way limits the possible uses of a crystal, which may be valuable in many different placements and situations.

MOHS SCALE

• **TALC (1):** The softest mineral, scratched by every other mineral and easily marked with a fingernail.

• **GYPSUM (2)**: Can be scratched with a fingernail using a greater pressure than 1. (A fingernail will mark any mineral with a hardness below 2.5.)

• **CALCITE (3)**: Can be scratched by a sharp coin.

• **FLOURITE (4)** Can be scratched with a penknife blade.

• **APATITE (5)**: Can be scratched with a difficulty using a steel point.

• **FELDSPAR (6)**: Will easily scratch glass.

• **QUARTZ (7)**: Will scratch most common surfaces.

• **TOPAZ (8):** Can scratch quartz.

• **CORUNDUM (9)**: Easily scratches topaz and quartz.

• **DIAMOND (10):** The hardest natural substance.

MALACHITE

CHEMICAL FORMULA: $Cu_2Co_3(OH)_2$
CRYSTAL SYSTEM: *Monoclinic*
HARDNESS: *3.5–4*
LUSTER: *Adamantine, silky, dull*
COLOR: *Green with dark green or black layers*
CHAKRA: *Heart*
SUBTLE BODY: *Etheric, emotional*

Malachite draws out emotional imbalances. It is especially protective from environmental pollutants to the heart chakra and the physical body. It will need regular cleansing; avoid salt, which damages the surface.

RUBY

CHEMICAL FORMULA: $Al_2O_3(+Cr)$
CRYSTAL SYSTEM: *Trigonal*
HARDNESS: *9*
LUSTER: *Vitreous to adamantine*
COLOR: *Red*
CHAKRA: *Heart*
SUBTLE BODY: *Mental, spiritual*

Ruby balances the heart at every level. It can enhance the physical function and the circulatory system. Confidence, security, self-esteem, and positive states of mind are increased.

AMBER

CHEMICAL FORMULA: $C_{10}H_{16}O + H_2S$
CRYSTAL SYSTEM: *Amorphous*
HARDNESS: *2*
LUSTER: *Resinous*
COLOR: *Yellow, brown, red, or green*
CHAKRA: *Solar plexus*
SUBTLE BODY: *Mental*

Amber helps warm and enliven. It is an excellent aid for nervous disorders and in detoxification.

SELENITE

CHEMICAL FORMULA: $CaSO_4.2H_2O$
CRYSTAL SYSTEM: *Monoclinic*
HARDNESS: *2*
LUSTER: *Vitreous to pearl*
COLOR: *Transparent, white, yellow, brown, red, or blue-gray*
CHAKRA: *Sacral, throat, crown*
SUBTLE BODY: *Emotional, soul, spiritual*

One of the very best shifters of energy, selenite can remove negativity from the auric field rapidly. The quality of frictionless flow, and rapid cooling and organizing energy, means that selenite is excellent at removing blocked and stagnant energy. It brings clarity to the mind and expands consciousness. Selenite is extremely soft and easily scratched by a fingernail, so gem-quality stones need careful handling. The crystals are also extemely sensitive to water and humidity. They will bend even when held in the hand and may slide apart and disintegrate in water.

CALCITE

CHEMICAL FORMULA: $CaCO_3$
CRYSTAL SYSTEM: *Hexagonal*
HARDNESS: *3*
LUSTER: *Vitreous, pearl, silky*
COLOR: *Colorless, allochromatic, black, blue, gray, brown, green, yellow, or red*
CHAKRA: *All*

Calcite of the appropriate color can clear and energize all the chakras. It has a fast, multidirectional quality and is a good remover of stagnant energy. It can easily shift levels of awareness. Both spheres and eggs are useful meditation tools.

PERIDOT

CHEMICAL FORMULA: $(Mg, Fe)_2 SiO_4$
CRYSTAL SYSTEM: *Orthorhombic*
HARDNESS: *6.5–7*
LUSTER: *Vitreous to greasy*
COLOR: *Yellow-green*
CHAKRA: *Heart, solar plexus*
SUBTLE BODY: *All*

An effective cleansing stone, said to be able to gradually remove all toxins from the body. It increases clarity of mind and optimism. It can help with visualization skills.

EMERALD
CHEMICAL FORMULA: *Be₃Al₂Si₆O₁₈*
CRYSTAL SYSTEM: *Hexagonal*
HARDNESS: *7.5–8*
LUSTER: *Vitreous*
COLOR: *Bright- green*
CHAKRA: *Heart*
SUBTLE BODY: *Etheric, emotional, astral*
A stone of harmony, emerald encourages peaceful growth and abundance. The heart chakra is strengthened by it.

FLUORITE
CHEMICAL FORMULA: *CaF₂*
CRYSTAL SYSTEM: *Cubic*
HARDNESS: *4*
COLOR: *Purple, blue, green, yellow, or clear*
LUSTER: *Vitreous*
CHAKRA: *Brow*
SUBTLE BODY: *Etheric*
Fluorite supports healthy bone tissue and physical structures of all organs. This stone helps balance coordination at physical levels, so it is useful for improving learning skills, dexterity, and balance.

PEARL
CHEMICAL FORMULA: *CaCO₃ + conchiolin + H₂O*
CRYSTAL SYSTEM: *Amorphous, orthorhombic*
HARDNESS: *2.5–3.5*
LUSTER: *Pearl*
COLOR: *White, pink, brown, or black*
CHAKRA: *Sacral, solar plexus*
SUBTLE BODY: *Etheric, emotional*
Pearl can balance the emotions and increase tolerance and flexibility. It influences aspects of solar plexus function, such as balance of physical energy, assimilation of nutrients, and self-assurance.

AMETRINE

Ametrine works well with headaches, tension, and stress-related illnesses, such as digestive upset and ulcers, balancing the energies of the solar plexus and the head. Ametrine also combines insight with clear thinking, so this is a useful stone for study. (See also: Citrine, Amethyst.)

RHODONITE

CHEMICAL FORMULA: $MnSiO_3$
CRYSTAL SYSTEM: *Triclinic*
HARDNESS: *5.5–6.5*
LUSTER: *Vitreous*
COLOR: *Pink to dark pink with brown or black areas*
CHAKRA: *Heart*
SUBTLE BODY: *Emotional*
Said to be useful for those people using mantras, increasing the meditation's effectiveness. Its color, like many pink stones, suggests a balancing of the heart chakra. It is a remedy for negative states, such as anxiety.

INDICOLITE
(BLUE TOURMALINE)

CHEMICAL FORMULA: $Na(Mg,Fe,Li,Mn,Al)3Al_6(BO_3)Si_6O_{18}(OH,F)_4$
CRYSTAL SYSTEM: *Trigonal*
HARDNESS: *7.5*
LUSTER: *Vitreous*
COLOR: *Blue, blue-green*
CHAKRA: *Throat, brow*
SUBTLE BODY: *All*
Indicolite works well with the throat center and its associated organs—the thyroid gland, lungs, larynx, and bones of the neck. Deep blue varieties activate the properties of the brow chakra, increasing the flow of information and intelligence.

COPPER

CHEMICAL FORMULA: *Cu*
CRYSTAL SYSTEM: *Cubic*
HARDNESS: *2.5–3*
LUSTER: *Metallic*
COLOR: *Copper, red*
CHAKRA: *Base, sacral, solar plexus, heart*
SUBTLE BODY: *All*

Copper's main action is to reduce inflammation, and it is well known as an aid to rheumatism and arthritis. It is strengthening on every level and helps the flow of energy, especially in the nervous system.

KUNZITE

CHEMICAL FORMULA: *LiAlSi$_2$O$_6$*
CRYSTAL SYSTEM: *Monoclinic*
HARDNESS: *6.5–7.5*
LUSTER: *Vitreous*
COLOR: *Pink, lilac pink (spodumene: clear; hiddenite: green)*
CHAKRA: *Heart, throat*
SUBTLE BODY: *Etheric*

A heart chakra cleanser and protector, kunzite can help remove negativity and create a meditative space. It also helps with the cardiovascular system and thyroid problems. It enhances life energy and self-esteem.

JASPER

CHEMICAL FORMULA: *SiO$_2$*
CRYSTAL SYSTEM: *Trigonal*
HARDNESS: *7*
LUSTER: *Dull to vitreous*
COLOR: *Red, yellow, green, blue, or brown*
CHAKRA: *Base, sacral, solar plexus, heart*
SUBTLE BODY: *Etheric*

Jasper is an earthy, grounding stone. The red variety is energizing and can be used to ground the base chakra. Other varieties will work with other chakras: yellow with the solar plexus; green with the heart.

SCHORL (BLACK TOURMALINE)

CHEMICAL FORMULA:
Na(Mg,Fe,Li,Mn,Al)$_3$Al$_6$(BO3)Si$_6$O$_{18}$(OH,F)$_4$
CRYSTAL SYSTEM: *Trigonal*
HARDNESS: *7–7.5*
LUSTER: *Vitreous*
COLOR: *Black*
CHAKRA: *Base*
SUBTLE BODY: *Etheric, astral*

An effective grounding stone, schorl stabilizes the energy of the base chakra. It realigns the bones and can help pulled and strained muscles. It is a useful protecting stone.

BLOODSTONE

CHEMICAL FORMULA: *SiO_2*
CRYSTAL SYSTEM: *Trigonal (microcrystalline)*
HARDNESS: *7*
LUSTER: *Vitreous*
COLOR: *Green with red spots*
CHAKRA: *Heart, base*
SUBTLE BODY: *Etheric*

Bloodstone can be used in healing where blood and circulation need support. It is a good physical energizer and motivator. It also helps bring spiritual qualities into practical everyday life.

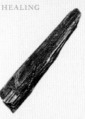

KYANITE

CHEMICAL FORMULA: *Al_2SiO_5*
CRYSTAL SYSTEM: *Triclinic*
HARDNESS: *4–7 (depending on direction)*
LUSTER: *Pearl, vitreous*
COLOR: *Blue, blue-black*
CHAKRA: *Throat*
SUBTLE BODY: *All*

Kyanite can be used to balance all chakras and subtle bodies. It brings calm and tranquility.

AGATE

CHEMICAL FORMULA: *SiO_2*
CRYSTAL SYSTEM: *Trigonal*
HARDNESS: *6.5*
LUSTER: *Vitreous*
COLOR: *Variegated colors in concentric bands*

Agate has a strengthening effect on the subtle anatomy and will help clarify and reveal underlying levels of information. Agate can be a useful meditation tool and is used in absent healing.

GARNET

CHEMICAL FORMULA: *$X_3Y_2(SiO_4)_3$*
where X = Calcium, iron, manganese, or magnesium and
Y = Chromium, aluminum, iron, or titanium
CRYSTAL SYSTEM: *Cubic*
HARDNESS: *6.5–7.5*
LUSTER: *Vitreous*
COLOR: *Red, brown, orange, or green*
CHAKRA: *Mostly base*
SUBTLE BODY: *Etheric, astral*

Red garnets are fine energizing stones. They will accelerate and amplify the actions of other nearby stones. The actions depend on stone color but will always focus energy toward practical support.

LABRADORITE

CHEMICAL FORMULA: *(Na, Ca)Al$_{1.2}$Si$_{3.2}$O$_8$*
CRYSTAL SYSTEM: *Triclinic*
HARDNESS: *6–6.5*
LUSTER: *Vitreous*
COLOR: *Gray with iridescence of green, yellow, orange, and peacock blue*
CHAKRA: *All*
SUBTLE BODY: *All*

With labradorite, ideas and intuitive knowledge are easy to access. It is a good stone to use for seeing new solutions and opportunities in life. It can work with every chakra and subtle body and is one of the best stones for protecting the aura.

SMOKY QUARTZ

CHEMICAL FORMULA: *SiO$_2$*
CRYSTAL SYSTEM: *Trigonal*
HARDNESS: *7*
LUSTER: *Vitreous*
COLOR: *Brown, smoky gray, or black*
CHAKRA: *Base, sacral, solar plexus*
SUBTLE BODY: *Emotional, mental, astral*

An effective, gentle grounding stone. It is quietening and calming with an even energy that can regulate and temper crystals of a more volatile nature. It will gently dissolve negative states of mind. It absorbs energy and information, giving protection to the whole being, both physical and emotional.

CARNELIAN

CHEMICAL FORMULA: *SiO$_2$*
CRYSTAL SYSTEM: *Trigonal*
HARDNESS: *7*
LUSTER: *Vitreous*
COLOR: *Red-orange*
CHAKRA: *Sacral*
SUBTLE BODY: *Etheric*

Gently warming, carnelian is a good all-round healing stone. It works well with the sacral chakra. It can be used together with other cooler stones to regulate the energy.

AMETHYST

CHEMICAL FORMULA: *SiO$_2$*
(quartz variety) + Fe (iron)
CRYSTAL SYSTEM: *Trigonal*
HARDNESS: *7*
LUSTER: *Vitreous*
COLOR: *Violet*
CHAKRA: *Brow, crown*
SUBTLE BODY: *Emotional, mental, spiritual*

A wonderful healing stone focused on calming and stabilizing. It can be used effectively as a meditation stone and works well with the brow and crown chakras.

MAGNETITE (AND LODESTONE)

CHEMICAL FORMULA: Fe_3O_4
CRYSTAL SYSTEM: *Cubic*
HARDNESS: *5.5–6.5*
LUSTER: *Metallic, dull*
COLOR: *Black*
CHAKRA: *All*
SUBTLE BODY: *All*

Excellent balancers of the energy systems, both stones can temporarily align the actions of all the chakras and subtle bodies, allowing the release of stress. The more obvious magnetism of lodestone stimulates the electrical properties of the body.

TOPAZ

CHEMICAL FORMULA: $Al_2SiO_4 (F.OH)_2$
CRYSTAL SYSTEM: *Orthorhombic*
HARDNESS: *8*
LUSTER: *Vitreous*
COLOR: *Orange, pink, yellow, white, blue, gray, green, brown, or clear*
CHAKRA: *Solar plexus*
SUBTLE BODY: *Etheric*

Topaz relaxes tension and helps stabilize the emotions. The energy of golden topaz works well with the crown chakra.

MOLDAVITE

CHEMICAL FORMULA: *Various silicates*
CRYSTAL SYSTEM: *Amorphous*
HARDNESS: *5*
LUSTER: *Vitreous*
COLOR: *Green*
CHAKRA: *Heart, throat, brow, crown*
SUBTLE BODY: *All higher bodies*

Moldavites are excellent amplifiers of other stones. They encourage the development of subtle senses, intuition, and an appreciation of the scale and beauty of creation. They work well with the heart, throat, brow, and crown chakras. If you are sensitive to the expansive heat of this stone, make sure you have a grounding stone nearby. Try it with celestite, danburite, sugilite, or apophyllite.

HEMATITE

CHEMICAL FORMULA: Fe_2O_3
CRYSTAL SYSTEM: *Trigonal*
HARDNESS: *5–6*
LUSTER: *Metallic or dull*
COLOR: *Metallic gray/black or red*
CHAKRA: *Sacral and solar plexus*
SUBTLE BODY: *Etheric*
One of the most effective grounding stones. Its high iron content supports the circulatory system and blood, as well as temperature regulation. It energizes the physical levels.

TOURMALINE

CHEMICAL FORMULA:
$Na(Mg, Fe, Li, Mn, Al)_3 Al_6 (BO_3) Si_6 O_{18} (OH, F)_4$
CRYSTAL SYSTEM: *Trigonal*
HARDNESS: *7–7.5*
LUSTER: *Vitreous*
COLOR: *Red, pink, yellow, green, blue, violet, black, multicolored, or colorless*
CHAKRA: *All*
SUBTLE BODY: *All*
All tourmalines have a powerful healing effect, harmonizing the subtle systems. Multicolored stones are ideal for the heart chakra; cat's eye and tourmaline quartz can be used at the brow and crown chakras.

CHRYSOPRASE

CHEMICAL FORMULA: SiO_2
CRYSTAL SYSTEM: *Trigonal*
HARDNESS: *7*
LUSTER: *Resinous to vitreous*
COLOR: *Apple green*
CHAKRA: *Heart, sacral*
SUBTLE BODY: *Etheric*
This mineral has been found useful for insomnia. It is deeply calming, both physically and emotionally, and may also be of use where there are sexual difficulties.

MOSS AGATE

CHEMICAL FORMULA: SiO_2
CRYSTAL SYSTEM: *Trigonal*
HARDNESS: *6.5*
LUSTER: *Vitreous to greasy*
COLOR: *Clear with green and brown inclusions*
CHAKRA: *Heart*
SUBTLE BODY: *Emotional, mental*
Moss agate helps establish personal space and the possibility of expansion and growth. It can free congested areas by acting on the lymphatic system. It increases optimism and helps encourage the desire to explore and experience more of life.

BLUE QUARTZ

CHEMICAL FORMULA: SiO_2
CRYSTAL SYSTEM: *Trigonal*
HARDNESS: *6.5–7*
LUSTER: *Vitreous to waxy*
COLOR: *Blue, blue-gray*
CHAKRA: *Throat, heart*
SUBTLE BODY: *All*

Works well with the organs and fuctions of the upper body. It can detoxify, cleanse, and repair.

OPAL

CHEMICAL FORMULA: SiO_2nH_2O
CRYSTAL STRUCTURE: *Amorphous*
HARDNESS: *6*
LUSTER: *Vitreous to pearl*
COLOR: *Various*
CHAKRA: *Mainly sacral, solar plexus, crown*
SUBTLE BODY: *Emotional body*

CHERRY OPAL SACRAL

Found in shades of pink, red, and orange, cherry opal is helpful in tissue regeneration, particularly with blood disorders. It gently increases energy levels and can help lift moods.

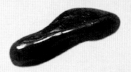

JADE

CHEMICAL FORMULA: $NaAlSi_2O_6$ (jadeite)
$Ca_2(Mg,Fe)_5Si_8O_{22}(OH)_2$ (nephrite)
CRYSTAL SYSTEM: *Monoclinic*
HARDNESS: *7.6–6.5*
LUSTER: *Waxy to vitreous*
COLOR: *Allochromatic, colorless to rich-green*
CHAKRA: *Heart*
SUBTLE BODY: *Astral, emotional, etheric*

Jade is two distinct minerals: nephrite and jadeite. Jade is a useful stone for the heart chakra. It helps stabilize and integrate the personality.

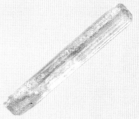

AQUAMARINE

CHEMICAL FORMULA: $Be_3Al_2Si_6O_{18}$
CRYSTAL SYSTEM: *Hexagonal*
HARDNESS: *7.5–8*
LUSTER: *Vitreous*
COLOR: *Blue*
CHAKRA: *Throat*
SUBTLE BODY: *Etheric, mental*

An excellent booster for the immune system. It works well with the thymus and throat areas. It encourages optimism and inspiration and can be helpful with creative expression.

COMMON OPAL

Common opal contains no iridescence or fire and can take on many colors, from milky white, gray, green, purple to brown, or clear. It has a more gentle energy than other opals and will focus its activity on the appropriate chakra color. Common opal stabilizes the emotions and feelings of self-worth. Common opal, like other varieties of opal, allows awareness of finer dimensional levels of reality.

WATER OPAL

Hyalite, also known as jelly opal or water opal, is a colorless, clear opal with rainbow colors and veils suspended within the stone. The ephemeral, other-worldly appearance of this gem can emphasize subtle, spiritual qualities of the emotions and the emotional body. It helps stabilize mood swings, eases the flow of life energy through the meridians and nadis, and makes a link between the sacral and crown chakras, which encourages enhanced meditative experiences.

WHITE OPAL

White opal is milky and is similar to common opal, although it does contain some colors. This stone is able to energize the crown chakra and bring clarity to the mind and a still calmness where necessary. Opals with an interplay of colors express and balance the energies of the crown chakra extremely well.

DARK OPAL

Dark-colored opals of brown, black, or gray-blue activate and balance the energies of the sacral chakra. It has been found to be one of the best stones to help premenstrual tension or menstrual cramps, bringing almost immediate relief when held or placed in a hip pocket. All opals work well at bringing emotional balance, and this variety will help with all sorts of sexual tension that has an emotional basis. Sensitivity is increased, and newly released emotions are assimilated.

DENDRITIC, OR TREE, OPAL

An opaque, common opal with impurities that form mosslike patterns. It can help patterns of growth, and the ability to organize and plan. All physical systems with branching structures like lungs, nerves, and blood can be helped, especially when constriction is present. Tree opals also connect well with nature.

FIRE OPAL

Fire opals are deep orange and red in color. An energizing, warming stone, it encourages recovery after emotional upsets and burnout or draining situations. Like all opals, fire opal works well with the fluid systems of the body and focuses on the emotional aspects of the self.

RHODOCHROSITE

CHEMICAL FORMULA: *$MnCO_3$*
CRYSTAL SYSTEM: *Trigonal*
HARDNESS: *3.5–4.5*
LUSTER: *Vitreous, pearl*
COLOR: *Pink, apricot, cream, or red*
CHAKRA: *Base, sacral, solar plexus, heart*
SUBTLE BODY: *Emotional, mental, astral*
Its main function is the stimulation and enhancement of self-worth and confidence, releasing tension from the emotional, mental, and astral bodies.

LAPIS LAZULI

CHEMICAL FORMULA: *$(Na, Ca)_8(Al.Si)_{12}O_{24}(S, SO_4)$*
CRYSTAL SYSTEM: *Cubic*
HARDNESS: *5.5*
LUSTER: *Vitreous to greasy*
COLOR: *Deep blues with white and gold*
CHAKRA: *Throat, brow*
SUBTLE BODY: *Etheric, mental*
Lapis lazuli works well with the throat and upper chest areas. It is an effective cleanser, drawing tension and anxiety from deep within the energy bodies. It activates every aspect of expression.

AZURITE

CHEMICAL FORMULA: *$Cu_3(CO_3)_2(OH)_2$*
CRYSTAL SYSTEM: *Monoclinic*
HARDNESS: *3.5–4*
LUSTER: *Vitreous, chalky*
COLOR: *Blue to dark- blue*
CHAKRA: *Throat, brow*
SUBTLE BODY: *Etheric, mental*
This stone can reach to deep levels of consciousness and draw out memories or old stresses. It stimulates all fine communication skills, creativity, and flow. It shifts all states toward integration and understanding.

BERYL

CHEMICAL FORMULA: *$Be_3Al_2Si_6O_{18}$*
CRYSTAL SYSTEM: *Hexagonal*
HARDNESS: *7–8*
LUSTER: *Vitreous*
COLOR: *Clear, yellow, pink, blue, or green*
CHAKRA: *All*
SUBTLE BODY: *All*
Beryl quietens the mind and helps relaxation, increasing calm, creativity, and self-worth. Bixbite (red) energizes the base chakra. Goshenite (colorless) helps the energy of the crown chakra. Morganite (pink) balances the heart chakra.

CITRINE

CHEMICAL FORMULA: *SiO₂, with inclusions*
CRYSTAL SYSTEM: *Trigonal*
HARDNESS: *7*
LUSTER: *Vitreous*
COLOR: *Yellow, golden brown, or orange-brown*
CHAKRA: *Solar plexus (sacral, base, crown)*
SUBTLE BODY: *Causal*

A warming, stimulating stone that is able to gently ground the base chakra, energize the second chakra with orange, or balance the yellow vibrations of the solar plexus.

BLUE LACE AGATE

CHEMICAL FORMULA: *SiO₂*
CRYSTAL SYSTEM: *Trigonal*
HARDNESS: *6.5*
LUSTER: *Vitreous to greasy*
COLOR: *Bands of blue, white, or gray*
CHAKRA: *Throat*
SUBTLE BODY: *Emotional, mental*

A cooling, calming stone that can be used anywhere where there is a buildup or excess of energy.

MOONSTONE

CHEMICAL FORMULA: *KAlSi₃O₈*
CRYSTAL SYSTEM: *Monoclinic*
HARDNESS: *6–6.5*
LUSTER: *Vitreous*
COLOR: *Pearly white, cream, yellow, or blue, sometimes with cat's eye or rainbows*
CHAKRA: *Sacral, solar plexus*
SUBTLE BODY: *Emotional*

An excellent stone for stabilizing the emotions and releasing tension. It can help disorders of the upper digestive tract, as well as menstrual cramps. It enhances intuition, creativity, and empathy.

QUARTZ

CHEMICAL FORMULA: *SiO₂*
CRYSTAL SYSTEM: *Trigonal*
HARDNESS: *7*
LUSTER: *Vitreous*
COLOR: *Transparent, white*
CHAKRA: *All*
SUBTLE BODY: *Etheric, emotional*

This stone amplifies and strengthens the whole auric field. It brings calm and clarity. It helps bring out the energy of stones placed nearby.

VERDELITE
(GREEN TOURMALINE)

CHEMICAL FORMULA:
$Na(Mg,Fe,Li,Mn,Al)3Al_6(BO_3)Si_6O_{18}(OH,F)_4$

CRYSTAL SYSTEM: *Trigonal*

HARDNESS: *7–7.5*

LUSTER: *Vitreous*

COLOR: *Green*

CHAKRA: *Heart*

SUBTLE BODY: *All*

Sometimes called Brazilian emerald, green tourmaline (verdelite) is a good balancer for the heart chakra. It also works well with the thymus gland and can strengthen the immune system. It will realign pulled and strained bone muscle and tissue. With it, there is a greater strengthening of the auric field to the energies of the planet, increasing confidence, security, and a sense of belonging.

TOURMALINE
QUARTZ

All colors of tourmaline can be found embedded in quartz, but the black variety, schorl, is the most common. Schorl is an effective grounding and protecting stone, closely linked to the planet's energies. It is one of the best stones for strengthening and protecting the subtle energy fields. Tourmaline quartz works well with the crown chakra energies. Order and coherence is given from the quartz, while the tourmaline grounds and deflects environmental disturbance.

RUTILE/ RUTILATED
QUARTZ

CHEMICAL FORMULA: TiO_2

CRYSTAL SYSTEM: *Tetragonal*

HARDNESS: *6–6.5*

LUSTER: *Adamantine, metallic*

COLOR: *Yellow, orange, deep red, or brown*

CHAKRA: *All*

SUBTLE BODY: *All*

An effective energy shifter, which is particularly useful for repairing torn and broken tissues. It can act as an integrator of all levels of energy.

RUBELLITE
(RED TOURMALINE)

CHEMICAL FORMULA: $Na(Mg,Fe,Li,Mn,Al)_3Al_6$ $(BO_3)Si_6O_{18}(OH,F)_4$

CRYSTAL SYSTEM: *Trigonal*

HARDNESS: *7–7.5*

LUSTER: *Vitreous*

COLOR: *Pink, red*

CHAKRA: *Sacral, heart*

SUBTLE BODY: *Emotional, astral*

Depending on the color, rubellite can be a stimulating or calming stone. In general, it balances the personality where there is too much aggression or passivity. It is energizing to the sacral chakra, increasing creativity.

GOLD

CHEMICAL FORMULA: *Au*
CRYSTAL SYSTEM: *Cubic*
HARDNESS: *2.5–3*
LUSTER: *Metallic*
COLOR: *Yellow, orange*
CHAKRA: *Heart*
SUBTLE BODY: *Emotional, mental, spiritual*

Gold balances the functions of the brain and nervous system and strengthens the immune system and major glands. It helps stabilize electrical functioning at cellular levels, reducing stress factors.

CELESTITE

CHEMICAL FORMULA: $SrSO_4$
CRYSTAL SYSTEM: *Orthorhombic*
HARDNESS: *3–3. 5*
LUSTER: *Vitreous to mother of pearl*
COLOR: *Clear, gray-blue, or sky blue*
CHAKRA: *Throat, crown*
SUBTLE BODY: *Soul*

Celestite has a cooling, uplifting energy that works well with the throat chakra, bringing lightness and relaxation. Inspiration, meditative states, and intuition align celestite to brow and crown chakras.

OBSIDIAN

CHEMICAL FORMULA: *Igneous rock containing feldspar, quartz, ilmenite, and magnetite*
HARDNESS: *6*
LUSTER: *Vitreous*
COLOR: *Black, greenish-black, gray, or red-brown*
CHAKRA: *Base, sacral, crown*
SUBTLE BODY: *Mental*

An effective grounding stone that can reveal deeply buried imbalances. It helps balance the digestive system, and to assimilate unacceptable truths.

SAPPHIRE

CHEMICAL FORMULA: Al_2O_3 (+Fe and Ti)
CRYSTAL SYSTEM: *Trigonal*
HARDNESS: *9*
LUSTER: *Subadamantine to vitreous*
COLOR: *Blue, violet-blue*
CHAKRA: *Solar plexus, heart, throat, crown*
SUBTLE BODY: *Emotional, astral*

Sapphire stimulates the higher mind and communication on subtle and spiritual levels. It is a calming, regulating stone, which helps balance the glandular system and eases tension.

AVENTURINE

CHEMICAL FORMULA: SiO_2, *with inclusions*
CRYSTAL SYSTEM: *Trigonal*
HARDNESS: *7*
LUSTER: *Vitreous*
COLOR: *Brown, green, or blue*
CHAKRA: *Heart*
SUBTLE BODY: *Etheric, emotional, mental*

This green stone promotes tranquility and a positive outlook and is an ideal stone for balancing the heart chakra. It helps stabilize the etheric, emotional, and mental bodies.

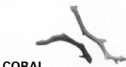

CORAL

CHEMICAL FORMULA: $CaCO_3$
CRYSTAL SYSTEM: *Hexagonal or trigonal*
HARDNESS: *3*
LUSTER: *Dull to vitreous*
COLOR: *Red, white, pink, golden, blue, or black*
CHAKRA: *Heart*
SUBTLE BODY: *Etheric*

Coral is an emotional balancer, with a positive value for the heart, blood, and circulatory systems.

SODALITE
CHEMICAL FORMULA: $Na_4Al_3Si_3O_{12}Cl$
CRYSTAL SYSTEM: *Cubic*
HARDNESS: *5.5–6*
LUSTER: *Vitreous to greasy*
COLOR: *Blue with white veining*
CHAKRA: *Throat, brow*
SUBTLE BODY: *Emotional, mental*
Sodalite works at the throat and brow chakras, where it clarifies perceptions and helps communication. It cools and stabilizes emotions, and works well with the lymphatic system, enhancing the immune system.

TIGER'S EYE
CHEMICAL FORMULA: SiO_2
CRYSTAL SYSTEM: *Trigonal*
HARDNESS: *7*
LUSTER: *Vitreous to silky*
COLOR: *Yellow to brown*
SUBTLE BODY: *Astral, causal*
This stone helps integrate the functions of the base, sacral, and solar plexus chakras, instilling confidence, practicality, and gentle grounding.

TURQUOISE
CHEMICAL FORMULA: $CuAl_6(PO_4)_4(OH)_{8.4-5}H_2O$
CRYSTAL SYSTEM: *Triclinic*
HARDNESS: *5–6*
LUSTER: *Waxy to vitreous*
COLOR: *Light blue*
CHAKRA: *All*
SUBTLE BODY: *All*
An all-purpose balancing and healing stone. It strengthens all the organs of the physical body, as well as the auric field, and will help repel environmental negativity. It has a natural connection to the spirit worlds.

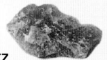

ROSE QUARTZ

CHEMICAL FORMULA: *SiO_2*
CRYSTAL SYSTEM: *Trigonal*
HARDNESS: *7*
LUSTER: *Vitreous*
COLOR: *Pink, rose, peach, or violet-pink*
CHAKRA: *Heart, throat*
SUBTLE BODY: *Emotional, mental, astral*
A powerful healing stone; small pieces can be calming and healing in all aggressive conditions. Personal issues, often at the root of emotional and mental tensions, can be eased with rose quartz.

SUGILITE

CHEMICAL FORMULA:
$KNa_2(Fe_2+,Mn_2+,Al)_2Li_3Si_{12}O_{30}$
CRYSTAL SYSTEM: *Hexagonal*
HARDNESS: *5.5–6.5*
LUSTER: *Vitreous to resinous*
COLOR: *Pink, lilac, or purple*
CHAKRA: *Crown*
SUBTLE BODY: *Astral, causal*
A useful healing tool for the crown chakra and the activities of the brain and nervous systems. It is effective where there is tension between spiritual and physical levels of reality.

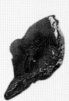

CHRYSOCOLLA

CHEMICAL FORMULA:
$Cu_2H_2Si_2O_5(OH)_4$
CRYSTAL SYSTEM: *Monoclinic or orthorhombic*
HARDNESS: *2–4*
LUSTER: *Vitreous to waxy*
COLOR: *Green, turquoise, or light to mid blues*
CHAKRA: *Heart, throat*
SUBTLE BODY: *Emotional, mental*
This stone's strong colors suggest effective use in the throat and chest areas. It is relaxing physically and emotionally.

Glossary

AFFIRMATIONS—Statements that emphasize positive states and emotions, helping remove self-limiting or erroneous beliefs or concepts.

ASTERISM—A star of light appearing on a crystal's surface caused by internal microcrystals. A true asterism will move around with a light source.

AURA—General term for the personal electromagnetic field and subtle bodies around the physical body.

CABOCHON—A method of cutting gemstones, usually semiprecious stones, with a flat oval base and a domed surface.

CENTERED/CENTERING—The state of being aware and focused within the physical body with a clear, calm mind.

CHAKRA—Spinning vortex of subtle energy.

CHATOYANCY—Play of light, silklike rippling, caused by light refracting off parallel microcrystals.

CHI—Chinese term for life energy flowing through the universe, concentrated within channels within the body.

CONCRETION—A mass of mineral matter found generally in a rock whose composition is different and produced by deposition from aqueous solution in the rock.

CRYSTAL—A mineral exhibiting regular planes and faces reflecting its internal organization of atoms.

CRYSTAL SYSTEM—A characteristic grouping of atoms that produce crystals with similar axes of symmetry and geometrical form.

DOUBLE-TERMINATED—A crystal that forms faceted points at both ends.

DOWSING—Various ways to access and indicate unconscious knowledge or sense data—for example, pendulum, rod, hand-scanning, muscle testing.

ELECTROMAGNETIC STRESS—Any strong field, either electrical or magnetic, that disrupts normal states within the body.

ENTRAINMENT—Where one system in a state of vibration or energy overrides another system's own vibrational frequency, causing resonance.

ESSENCES—Preparations of water charged with the energy signature of the gemstone, flower, or other object placed within it while exposed to sunlight.

GROUNDING—Techniques that allow excess and out-of-balance energies to flow from the body.

HOLISTIC—Viewing the body, mind, and emotions as an integrated system, in which change in one will affect the whole.

IGNEOUS—Rock formed from molten material. Called intrusive if it solidifies before reaching the Earth's surface.

INCLUSION—A solid foreign body enclosed in a mineral mass, often in the form of another crystalline mineral, gas, or water droplets.

INDICATOR MUSCLE—A muscle used in kinesiology, whose function shows a "yes" or "no" response to a question.

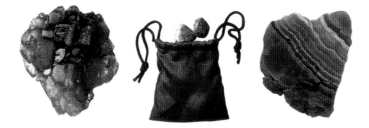

KINESIOLOGY—Also known as muscle testing. A way of assessing energy flow through muscle tone and correcting energy imbalances.

LATTICE—The regular pattern of atoms composing crystals' internal structure.

MATRIX—The base rock from which crystals grow.

MERIDIAN—Subtle energy channel running close to the surface of the skin, along which can be found sensitive places such as acupuncture points.

METAMORPHIC—A rock changed or modified by heat and pressure.

MINERAL—A single chemical compound. Minerals can be a single element such as diamond or a complex combination of atoms such as tourmaline.

NADIS—Nonphysical channels throughout the body carrying energy from each chakra.

RESONANCE—The effects of one system or body beginning to vibrate at the same rate as another already in a state of vibration. *See: Entrainment.*

ROCK—Sometimes a single mineral, most often a combination of different minerals and crystal structures.

SCHILLER—Twinkle or sparkle in a stone created by light reflecting off microcrystals.

SEDIMENTARY—Rock formed from layers of dust and fine material, compressed by its own weight and water.

SHAMAN—A general term for those skilled in working with the spirit worlds, particularly for healing and helping the tribal group.

STRONG-INDICATOR MUSCLE—The foundation of accurate muscle testing. A muscle that effortlessly resists gentle pressure.

SUBTLE BODY—Nonphysical aspects of consciousness that surround and interpenetrate the physical body.

SWITCHING—Where the meridian system becomes unstable through stress, making muscle testing unreliable.

TAPPING IN—Finger tapping around specific areas to bring the meridian system into balance. For grounding and centering.

TERMINATION—The natural end facets of a crystal, usually meeting in a point.

VIBRATIONAL HEALING—A general term for nonphysical healing modalities, including crystal healing, color healing, sound healing, and vibrational essences.

WITNESS—A link by which a healer assesses the energy state of a person not physically present, usually from a sample of hair, photograph, or signature.

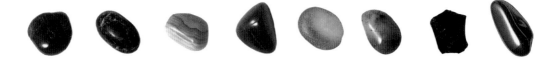

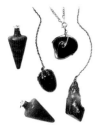

Further Reading and Useful Addresses

BAER, R. AND BAER, V.,
Windows of Light (Harper and Row, 1984)

BONEWITZ, R., *Cosmic Crystals*
(The Aquarian Press, 1983)

COWAN, D. AND GIRDLESTONE, R.,
Safe as Houses? (Gateway Books, 1996)

DIAMOND, J., *Life Energy*
(Dodd Mead & Co., 1985)

ELIADE, M., *Shamanism*
(Penguin, 1989)

GARDNER, J., *Color and Crystals*
(The Crossing Press, 1988)

GERBER, R., *Vibrational Medicine*
(Bear & Co., 1988)

GURUDAS, *Gem Elixirs and
Vibrational Healing*,
Vol. I (Cassandra Press, 1989)

JOHARI, H., *The Healing Power of
Gemstones* (Destiny Books, 1988)

JUDITH, A., *Wheels of Life*
(Llewellyn, 1987)

LILLY, S. AND LILLY, S., *Crystal Doorways*
(Capall Bann, 1997)

MELODY, *Love is in the Earth*
(Earth Love Publishing House, 1991)

PAULSON, G. L., *Kundalini and the Chakras*
(Llewellyn, 1991)

PAWLIK, J. AND CHASE, P., *The
Newcastle Guide to Healing with Crystals*
(Newcastle Publishing Co., 1988)

RAPHAELL, K., *Crystal Enlightenment*
(Aurora Press, 1985)

ROBINS, D., *The Secret Language of Stone*
(Rider, 1988)

SIBLAY, U., *The Complete Crystal Guidebook*
(Bantam, 1986)

TANSLEY, D., *Radionics and the Subtle
Anatomy of Man* (C.W. Daniel, 1972)

TANSLEY, D., *The Raiment of Light*
(Arkana, 1984)

EUROPE
Simon and Sue Lilly
Institute of Crystal and Gem Therapists
MCS P.O. Box 6
Exeter EX6 8YE
U.K.
+44 (0)1392 832005
Email: cgt@greenmantrees.demon.co.uk

**Affiliation of Crystal Healing
Organisations**
(Represents ten schools within the U.K.)
P.O. Box 100
Exminster
Exeter EX6 8YT
U.K.
+44(0)1479 841450
Email: acho@greentrees.demon.co.uk
www.crystal-healing.org

U.S.A.
**Crystal Academy of Advanced
Healing Arts**
(Katrina Raphael)
P.O. Box 1334
Kappa Kauai,
Hawaii 96746
U.S.A.
(001) 808 823 6959
www.webcrystalacademy.com

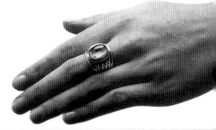

Index

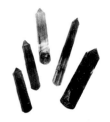

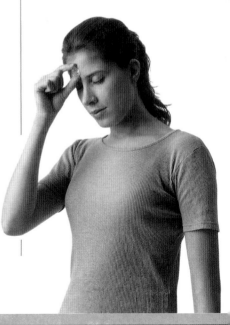

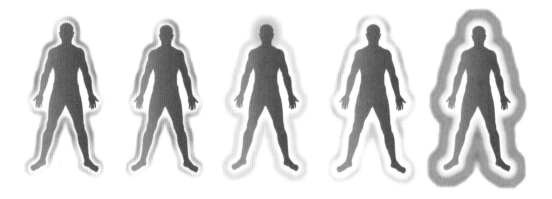

Picture Credits:

About the Author

SIMON LILLY has been a crystal therapist and color therapist for nearly twenty years. He has also studied different forms of kinesiology and the use of flower essences. With his wife Sue, he developed and produces 'Green Man Essences', a large range of vibrational essences gathered from British trees. He is a senior tutor at the Institute of Crystal and Gem Therapists (ICGT), which is a founder member of the Affiliation of Crystal Healing Organisations (ACHO). He has written over a dozen books on crystal healing, flower essences, and working with vibrational remedies. Simon lives and works in Devon, England.

Other Books in the Complete Illustrated Guide Series

The Complete Illustrated Guide to Massage

The Complete Illustrated Guide to Reflexology

The Complete Illustrated Guide to Natural Home Remedies

The Complete Illustrated Guide to Tai Chi

The Complete Illustrated Guide to Herbs

The Complete Illustrated Guide to Palmistry